THE COMPLETE
CORTISOL DETOX
DIET PLAN

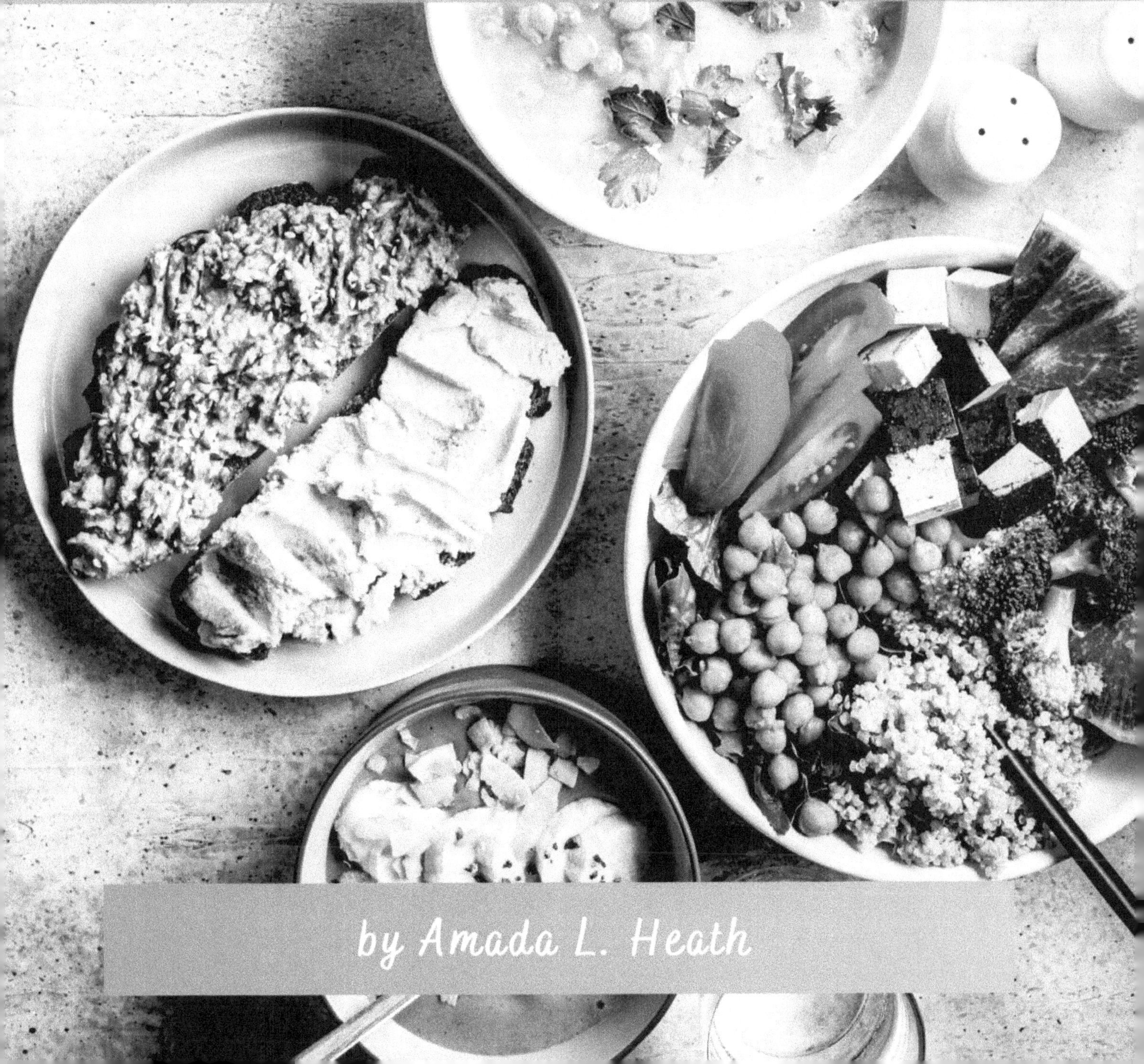

by Amada L. Heath

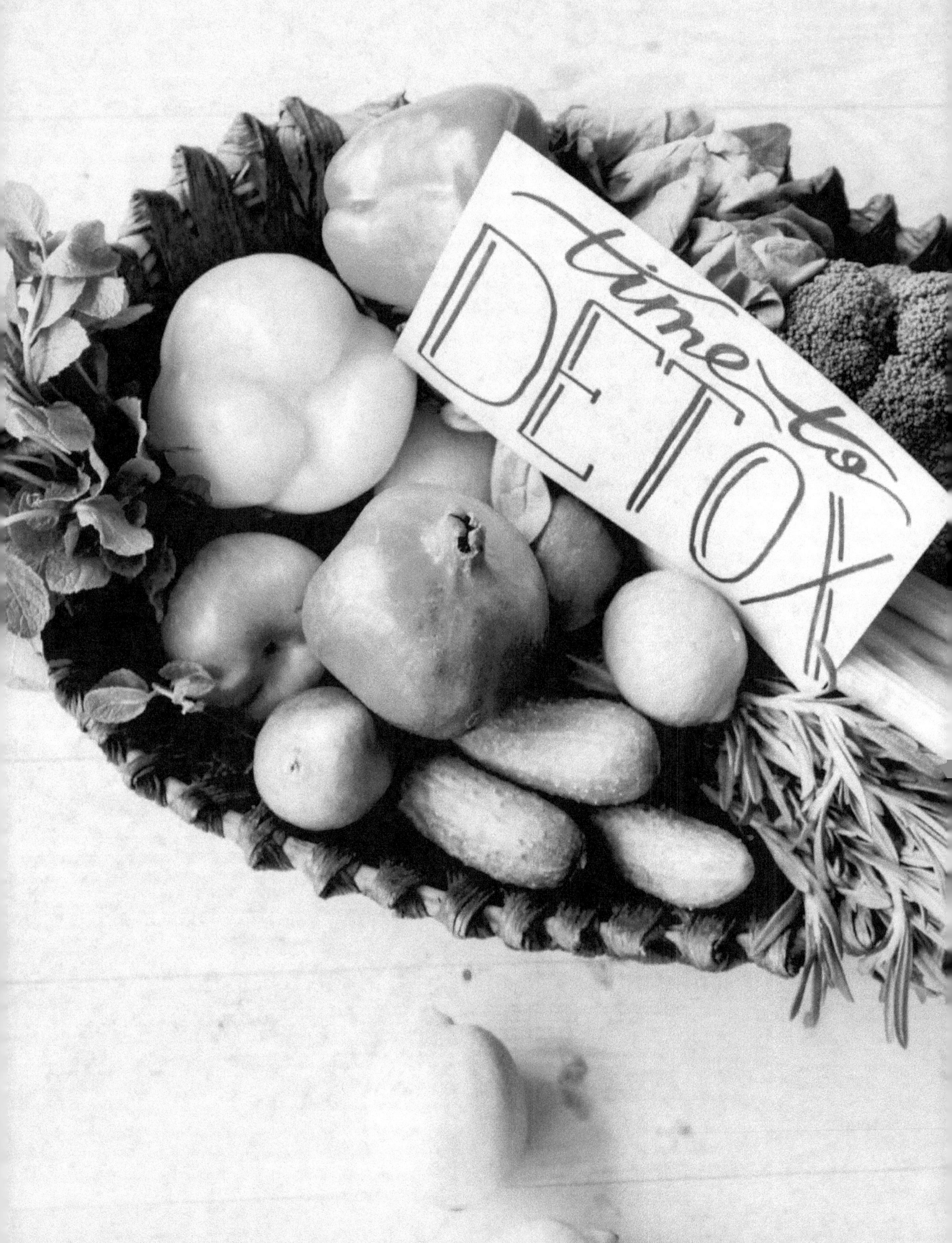

time to
DETOX

copyright

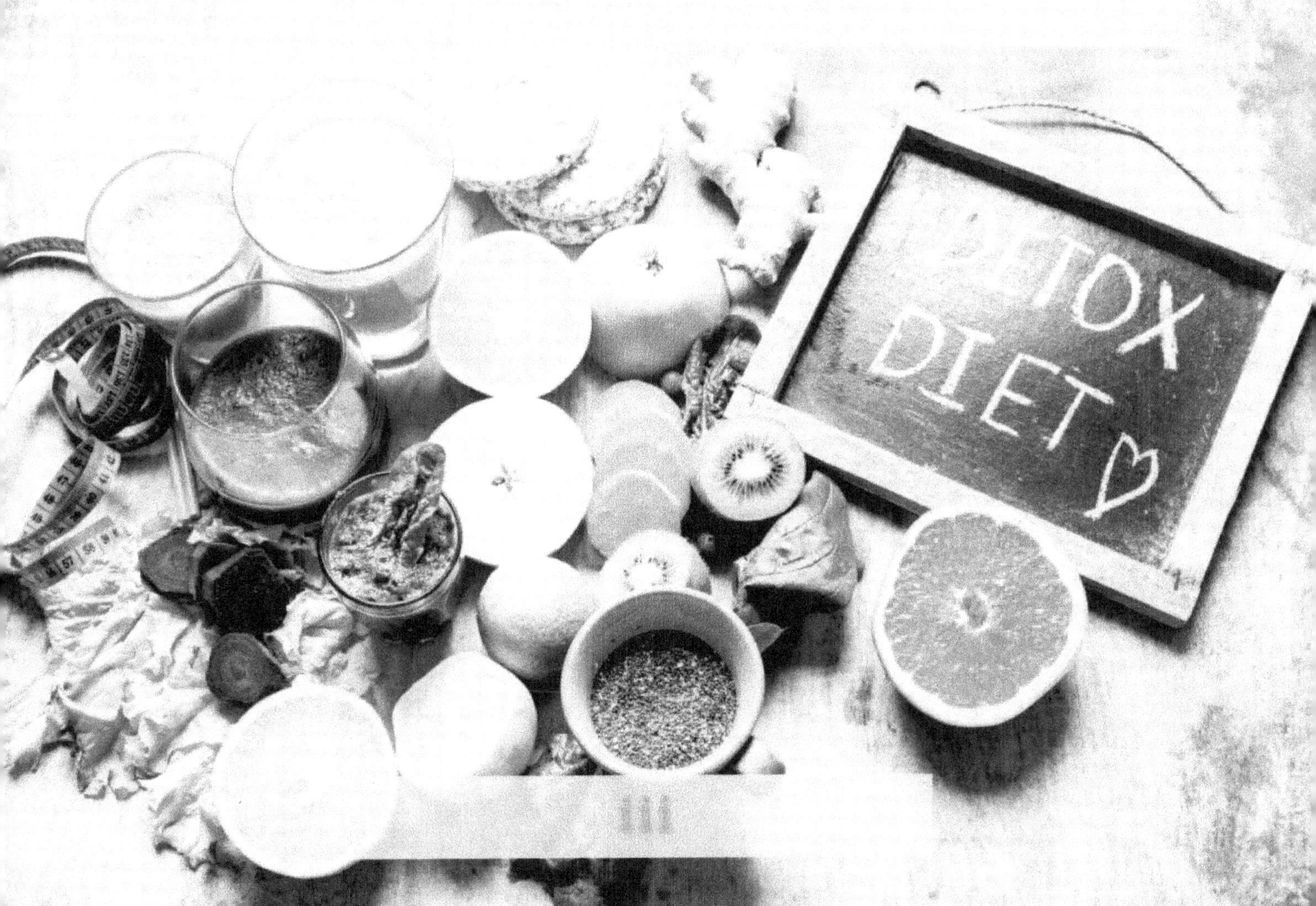

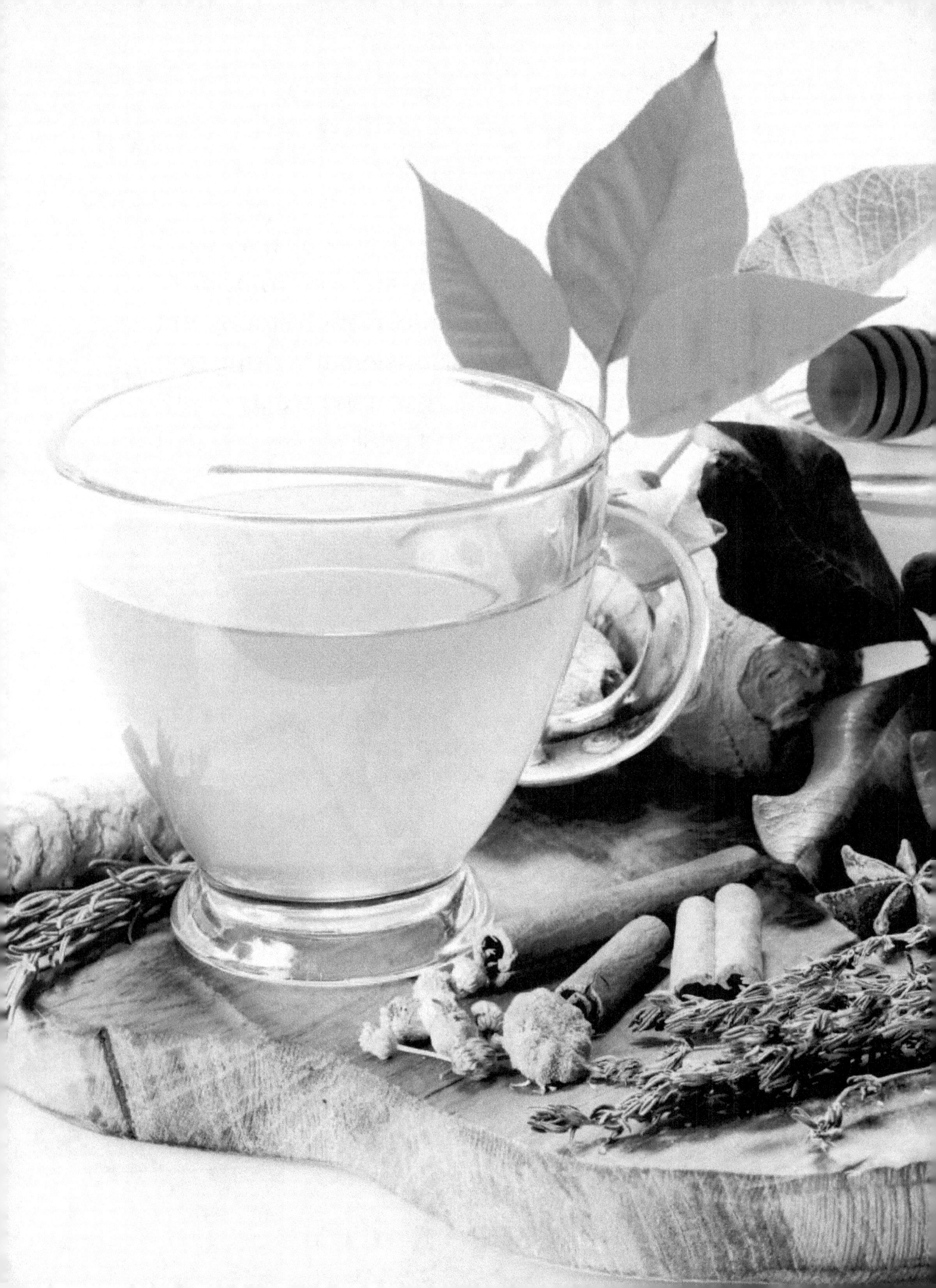

Table Of Contents

INTRODUCTION

In the small, peaceful town of Willow Creek lived Mary, an 68-year-old woman known for her vibrant energy and calm demeanor. Yet, only a few years ago, Mary struggled with chronic stress, anxiety, and fatigue that seemed to overshadow her zest for life.

Despite trying to stay active and lead a healthy lifestyle, she faced sleepless nights, persistent tiredness, and an overwhelming sense of stress that never seemed to leave her side. After a visit to her doctor, Mary discovered that her cortisol levels—the body's primary stress hormone—were out of balance, causing her to feel constantly on edge.

Mary decided to take control of her health, starting her journey with "The Complete Cortisol Detox Diet Plan." It wasn't just another diet; it was a comprehensive lifestyle change that aimed to restore balance to her body through mindful eating, proper exercise, sleep, and stress management.

Armed with knowledge, Mary incorporated nutrient-dense, anti-inflammatory foods, rich in omega-3s and antioxidants, and cut back on sugar and caffeine, which had been spiking her cortisol levels. She started her mornings with nourishing breakfasts like coconut chia seed pudding or savory avocado and egg toast.

Lunches were wholesome, including quinoa and bean salads, while dinners often featured balanced dishes like baked lemon herb chicken and sautéed shrimp with spinach. Each meal was thoughtfully designed to promote relaxation, improve gut health, and stabilize blood sugar.

But it wasn't just about food. Mary learned how to embrace meditation, yoga, and daily relaxation breaks to lower her stress and anxiety. Her nighttime routine shifted to prioritize restful sleep, with gentle stretches and chamomile tea helping her unwind.

Physical activity became a mindful practice, with nature walks replacing intense, stress-inducing workouts. She even made it a point to connect with loved ones regularly, sharing laughs, stories, and meals that brought joy and comfort.

Within weeks, Mary felt the transformation. Her energy returned, her sleep improved, and the heaviness of anxiety lifted, replaced by a sense of calm and balance. By managing cortisol naturally through diet, sleep, and stress-reducing habits, she had found the key to a healthier, happier life.

Today, Mary's journey inspires others to embark on their own path to balance, proving that even in the face of life's challenges, finding harmony with the right lifestyle choices can lead to a life filled with peace and well-being.

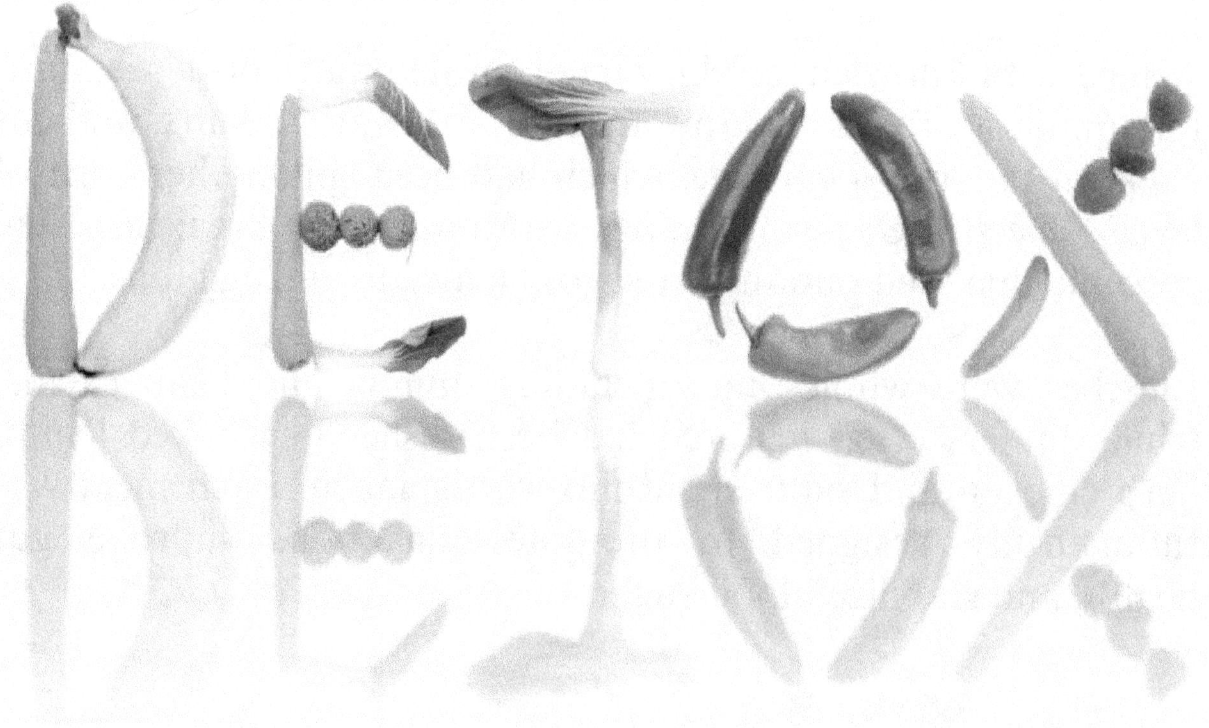

UNDERSTANDING CORTISOL

The Cortisol Diet revolves around managing the hormone cortisol, which plays a key role in the body's stress response. Cortisol, often called the "stress hormone," is produced by the adrenal glands and helps regulate metabolism, reduce inflammation, and assist in overall bodily functions, including controlling blood sugar levels and managing how the body utilizes carbohydrates, fats, and proteins. However, chronic stress and elevated cortisol levels can lead to weight gain, particularly in the abdominal area, muscle weakness, fatigue, anxiety, and other health issues. Therefore, the goal of a Cortisol Diet is to help balance and reduce excessive cortisol production through strategic nutrition,

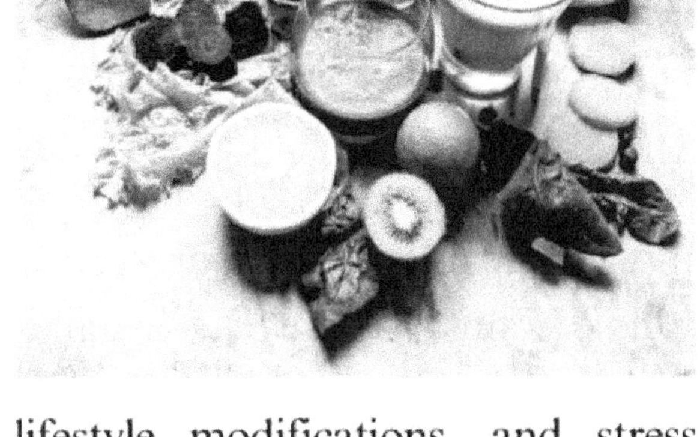

lifestyle modifications, and stress management.

"The Complete Cortisol Detox Diet Plan," the aim is to provide a structured program designed to support the body in effectively managing cortisol levels, detoxifying stress-induced toxins, and promoting overall health. This diet plan incorporates nutrient-dense foods, meal timing, and lifestyle strategies that aid in reducing stress, stabilizing energy, and enhancing the body's ability to recover from stress.

The plan often involves the following components:

1. Stress-Reducing Nutrition

The diet focuses on foods that naturally lower cortisol production and stress in the body. Consuming balanced meals with adequate protein, healthy fats, fiber, and complex carbohydrates helps regulate blood sugar levels, which is crucial in controlling cortisol.

Low glycemic index foods such as whole grains, leafy greens, legumes, berries, nuts, and seeds play a significant role in maintaining balanced energy and reducing the risk of cortisol spikes.

Foods rich in magnesium, vitamin C, B vitamins, and omega-3 fatty acids, like avocados, bananas, fatty fish, and dark chocolate, are emphasized for their stress-relieving properties.

2. Anti-Inflammatory Foods

Since cortisol is also associated with inflammation control, the diet plan aims to incorporate anti-inflammatory foods that can assist in reducing the overall inflammation in the body. Such foods

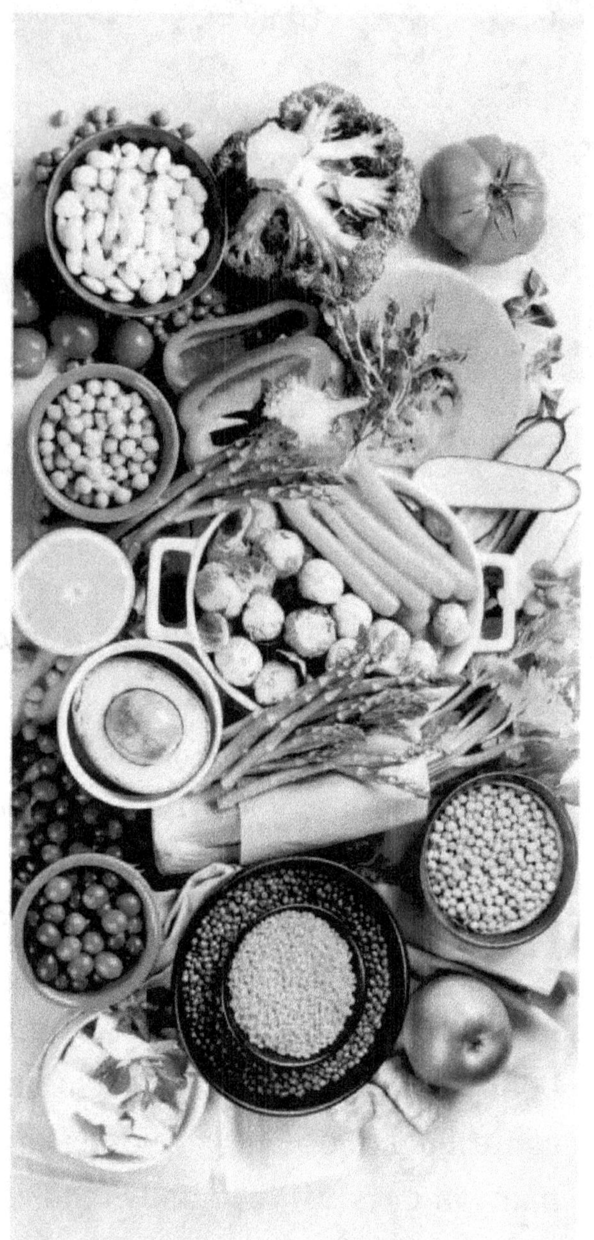

include leafy vegetables, fruits like berries and citrus, olive oil, nuts, seeds, and lean proteins. Reducing inflammation not only helps lower stress on the body but also improves immune function and digestive health, which are often compromised when cortisol is elevated.

The "Complete Cortisol Detox Diet Plan" often includes a focus on enhancing gut health since a healthy digestive system is crucial for nutrient absorption and hormone regulation.

Probiotics and prebiotic-rich foods such as yogurt, kefir, sauerkraut, kimchi, garlic, and onions are included to promote a healthy balance of gut bacteria. Supporting the liver, which plays a key role in detoxification, is also integral to the plan, achieved through foods like cruciferous vegetables (broccoli, cauliflower), herbs (turmeric, ginger), and adequate hydration. These foods help the body efficiently eliminate toxins that can exacerbate stress and disrupt cortisol balance.

Meal timing is another critical aspect of the Cortisol Detox Diet. Eating balanced meals at regular intervals, particularly not skipping breakfast, is crucial in maintaining stable blood sugar levels throughout the day, which directly influences cortisol regulation. Incorporating protein-rich snacks between meals helps to prevent energy dips and cortisol spikes. The plan may recommend reducing caffeine and sugar intake, particularly in the late afternoon and evening, to avoid disrupting the natural cortisol rhythm and sleep cycle.

Beyond just food choices, the diet plan incorporates lifestyle changes that support reducing overall stress and improving cortisol balance. Mindful eating practices, such as eating slowly, appreciating flavors, and avoiding distractions like screens during meals, can help reduce stress levels associated with eating habits.

Additionally, incorporating regular physical activity like yoga, moderate cardio, and strength training can be beneficial as exercise helps regulate cortisol, provided it's balanced and not excessive.

6. Stress Management and Sleep Hygiene

Managing stress is central to the Cortisol Diet, as stress is the primary trigger for increased cortisol levels. The plan includes strategies for stress management like meditation, breathing exercises, and hobbies that promote relaxation.

Adequate sleep is also emphasized, as poor sleep is closely linked to increased cortisol production. Recommendations might include setting a consistent sleep schedule, creating a calming nighttime routine, and reducing screen time before bed.

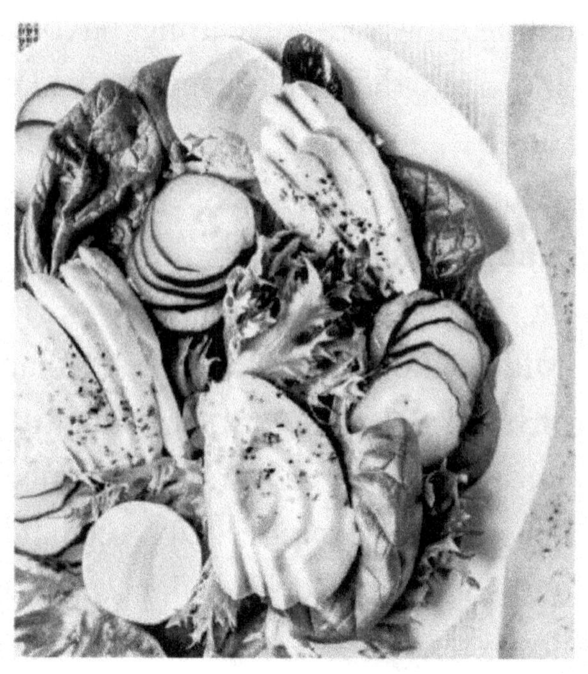

ROLE OF CORTISOL IN THE BODY

Cortisol is a crucial hormone produced by the adrenal glands that plays a significant role in the body's stress response, metabolism, immune function, and overall homeostasis. Known as the "stress hormone," cortisol is released in response to stress and low blood glucose levels. It is part of the body's "fight-or-flight" mechanism, helping to prepare the body to respond to perceived threats by increasing alertness, energy levels, and the availability of glucose.

Metabolic Regulation

Cortisol helps regulate the metabolism of fats, proteins, and carbohydrates. It promotes the breakdown of proteins into amino acids, which can be converted into glucose (gluconeogenesis), and also stimulates the release of fatty acids for energy use. This metabolic function is crucial for ensuring the body has enough energy, particularly during stress or fasting.

Cortisol helps maintain blood pressure by regulating the balance of salt and water in the body, which is essential for cardiovascular function.

It ensures that blood vessels respond effectively to hormones that constrict or dilate them, thereby contributing to proper circulation and maintaining adequate blood pressure levels.

Cortisol plays an anti-inflammatory role by suppressing the immune system's response to perceived threats, helping to reduce inflammation and allergic reactions.

While this helps to prevent overreactions to stress or injury, chronically high cortisol levels can lead to weakened immune function and increased susceptibility to infections.

Cortisol is released in greater amounts during stress to prepare the body for a "fight-or-flight" response.

It temporarily increases energy availability by raising blood glucose and enhancing tissue repair. However, when cortisol levels remain elevated over time due to chronic stress, it can lead to negative effects, such as anxiety, weight gain, impaired cognition, and disrupted sleep cycles.

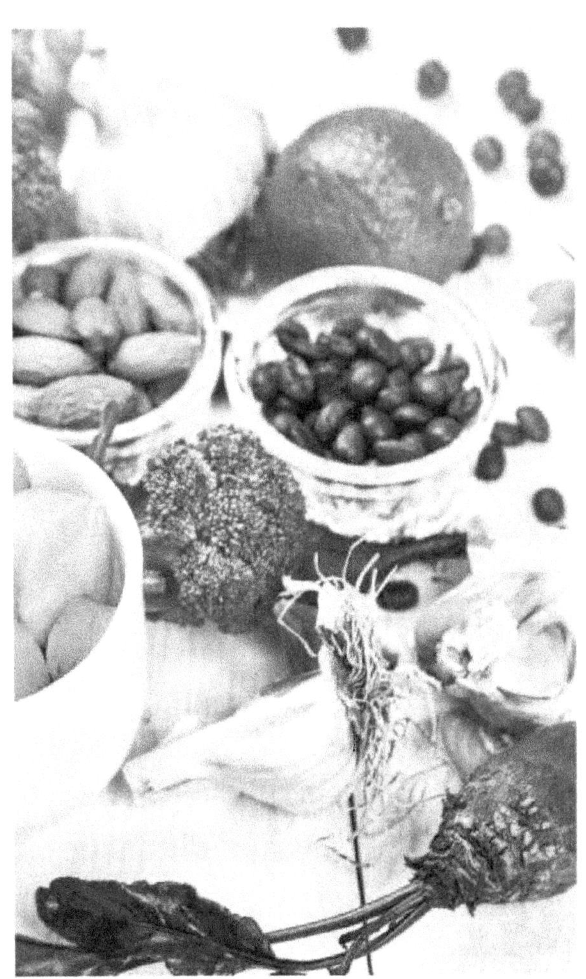

EFFECT OF CORTISOL ON THE MENTAL AND PHYSICAL HEALTH

Cortisol, while essential for normal body functions, can have several effects on both mental and physical health, especially when levels are chronically elevated due to prolonged stress.

Mental Health Effects:

Anxiety and Depression: Prolonged elevated cortisol levels can lead to increased feelings of anxiety and even contribute to depression. Cortisol can affect neurotransmitter balance, particularly serotonin and dopamine, which are crucial for mood regulation.

Memory and Cognitive Function:

High levels of cortisol can impair cognitive function, memory retention, and concentration. It can shrink the hippocampus, the brain area responsible for learning and memory, potentially leading to memory problems and difficulties in decision-making.

Mood Swings and Irritability:

Chronic cortisol elevation can result in mood swings, increased irritability, and emotional instability. This can affect relationships and day-to-day emotional well-being.

Sleep Disruption:

High cortisol levels, particularly in the evening, can interfere with the body's natural sleep-wake cycle (circadian rhythm). This can lead to difficulty falling asleep, poor sleep quality, and insomnia, further contributing to stress and mental fatigue.

Physical Health Effects:

Weight Gain and Obesity: Cortisol increases appetite and cravings for high-calorie foods, often leading to overeating and weight gain. It also promotes fat storage, particularly in the abdominal area, which is linked to metabolic issues.

Immune System Suppression: While cortisol has anti-inflammatory properties, chronic elevation can suppress the immune system, making the body more susceptible to infections and impairing its ability to recover from illness or injury.

High Blood Pressure and Cardiovascular Risk: Cortisol helps regulate blood pressure, but persistently high levels can lead to hypertension. Elevated cortisol can also contribute to an increased risk of heart disease, as it may lead to higher cholesterol and inflammation.

Muscle Weakness and Bone Density Loss: Cortisol can break down proteins and reduce bone formation, leading to muscle weakness and potential osteoporosis or decreased bone density over time.

Digestive Problems: Elevated cortisol levels can impact digestive health by increasing the risk of gastrointestinal issues such as irritable bowel syndrome (IBS) and ulcers. Stress often disrupts digestion and nutrient absorption.

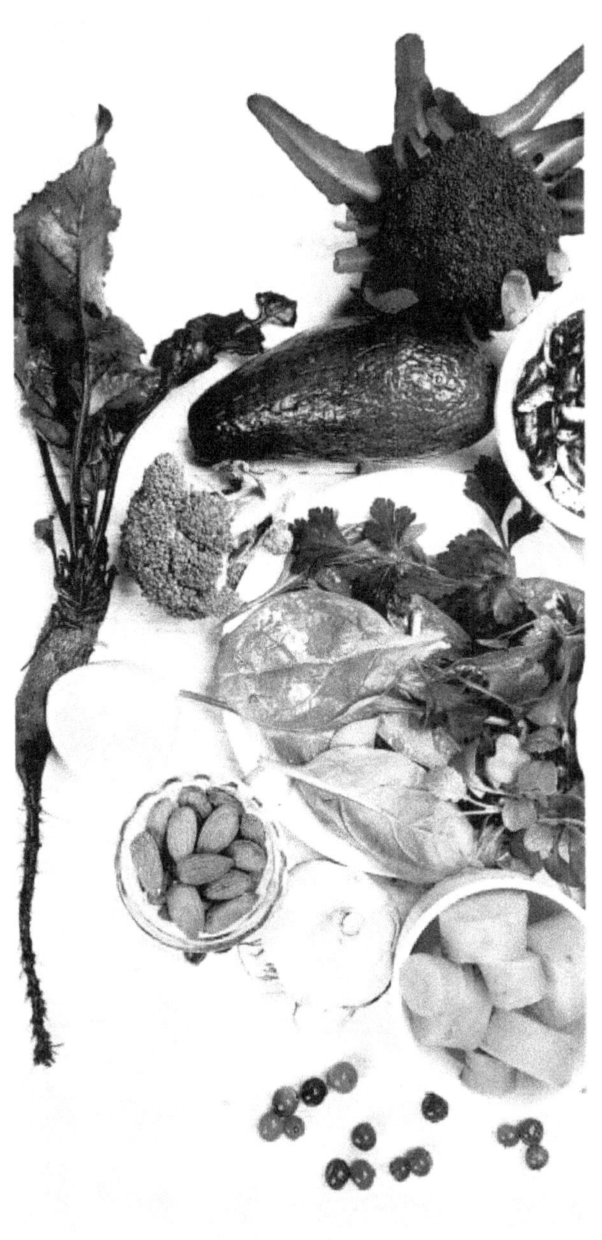

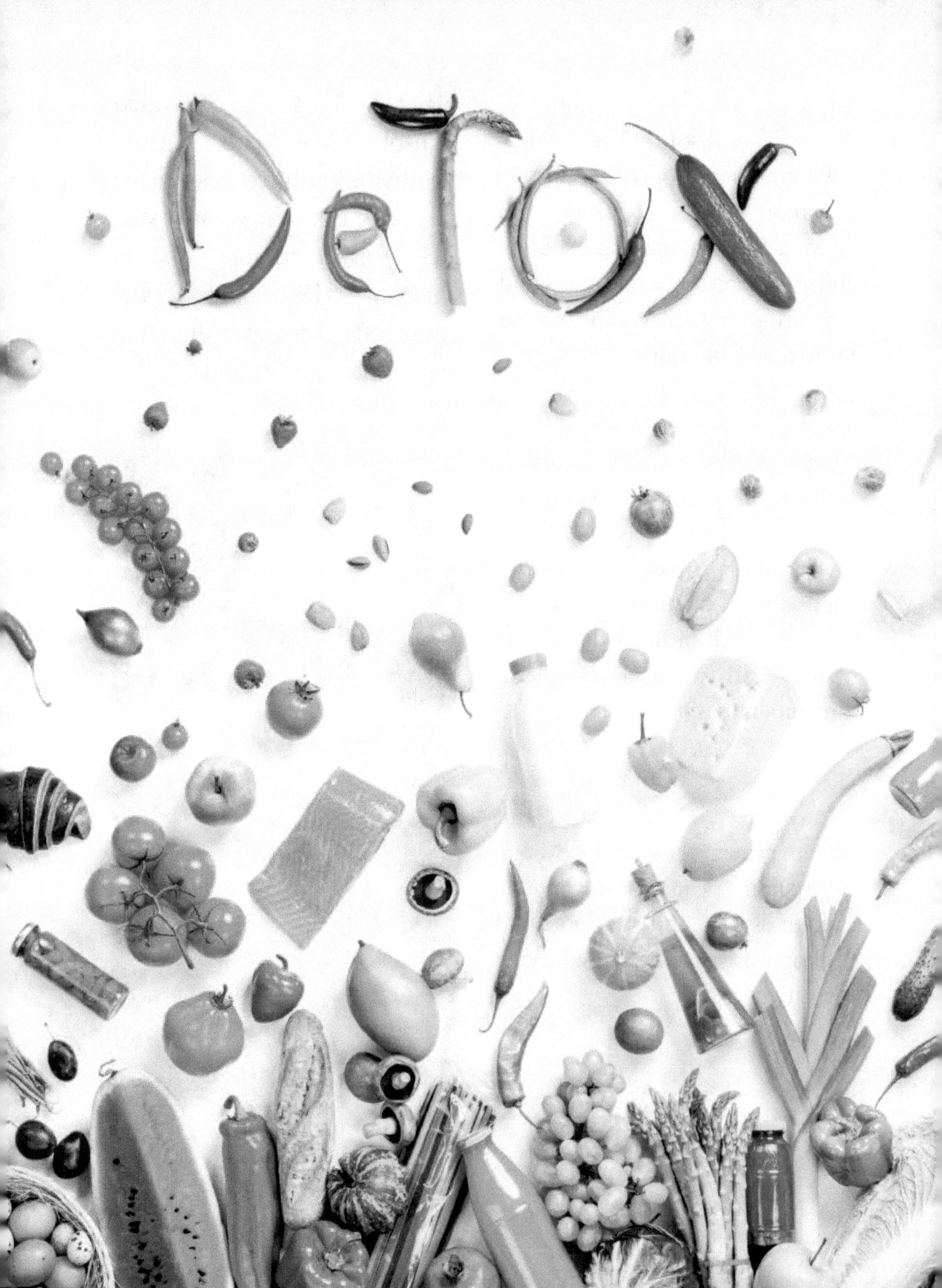
DeToX

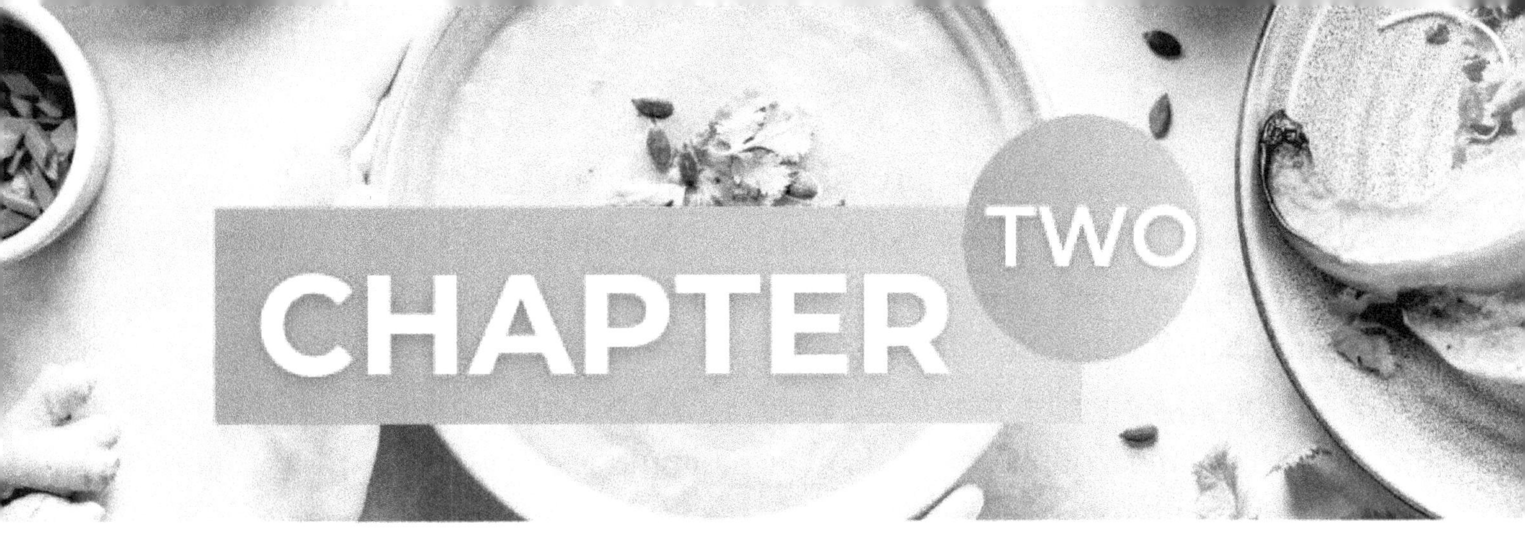

IMPORTANCE OF DETOXING CORTISOL

Detoxing cortisol is important for maintaining both mental and physical health, particularly in managing the adverse effects of chronic stress. Cortisol, known as the body's "stress hormone," is vital for various functions such as metabolism, immune response, and the regulation of the sleep-wake cycle.

However, prolonged high levels of cortisol due to chronic stress can harm the body and mind. Detoxifying cortisol means helping the body regulate and reduce excess levels, restoring hormonal balance, and preventing health complications.

1. Reducing Stress and Anxiety

Cortisol is released during stressful situations to prepare the body for a "fight-or-flight" response. While this is beneficial in short bursts, long-term stress leads to consistently elevated cortisol levels. This can cause anxiety, irritability, and difficulty coping with stressful situations. Detoxing cortisol through stress management techniques, a balanced diet, and lifestyle changes helps lower anxiety levels and promote a calmer mental state.

2. Enhancing Sleep Quality

Excess cortisol disrupts the body's natural sleep-wake cycle by keeping the body alert and awake. This often leads to difficulty falling asleep, poor-quality sleep, and insomnia. By detoxifying and lowering cortisol levels, the body can better regulate its circadian rhythm, leading to improved sleep quality and duration. Adequate sleep is vital for emotional resilience, cognitive function, and overall well-being.

3. Preventing Weight Gain and Improving Metabolism

Chronic elevated cortisol promotes fat storage, particularly in the abdominal area, and increases cravings for sugary and high-fat foods. This can contribute to obesity and metabolic disorders like type 2 diabetes. Detoxing cortisol helps to stabilize blood sugar levels, control cravings, and improve metabolism, making it easier to maintain a healthy weight and reduce the risk of obesity-related health issues.

4. Supporting Immune Function

While cortisol has anti-inflammatory properties and helps the immune system respond to threats, too much of it can suppress immune function over time.

This makes the body more vulnerable to infections, inflammation, and slower recovery from illnesses or injuries. Detoxifying cortisol allows the immune system to function optimally, reducing the risk of infections and improving the body's ability to fight off diseases.

5. Promoting Better Mental Clarity and Cognitive Health

High cortisol levels can impair memory, decision-making, and concentration by shrinking the hippocampus, the brain region responsible for learning and memory. This can lead to cognitive difficulties, brain fog, and impaired focus. By detoxing cortisol, cognitive function can improve, supporting sharper mental clarity, better memory retention, and enhanced problem-solving skills.

6. Balancing Hormones and Preventing Chronic Health Issues

Detoxifying cortisol is also crucial for balancing other hormones, such as insulin, thyroid hormones, and sex hormones like estrogen and testosterone. Chronic high cortisol levels can lead to hormonal imbalances, contributing to health conditions like adrenal fatigue, metabolic syndrome, hypothyroidism, and reproductive health issues. Detoxing cortisol helps maintain overall hormonal balance and prevents the onset of such chronic conditions.

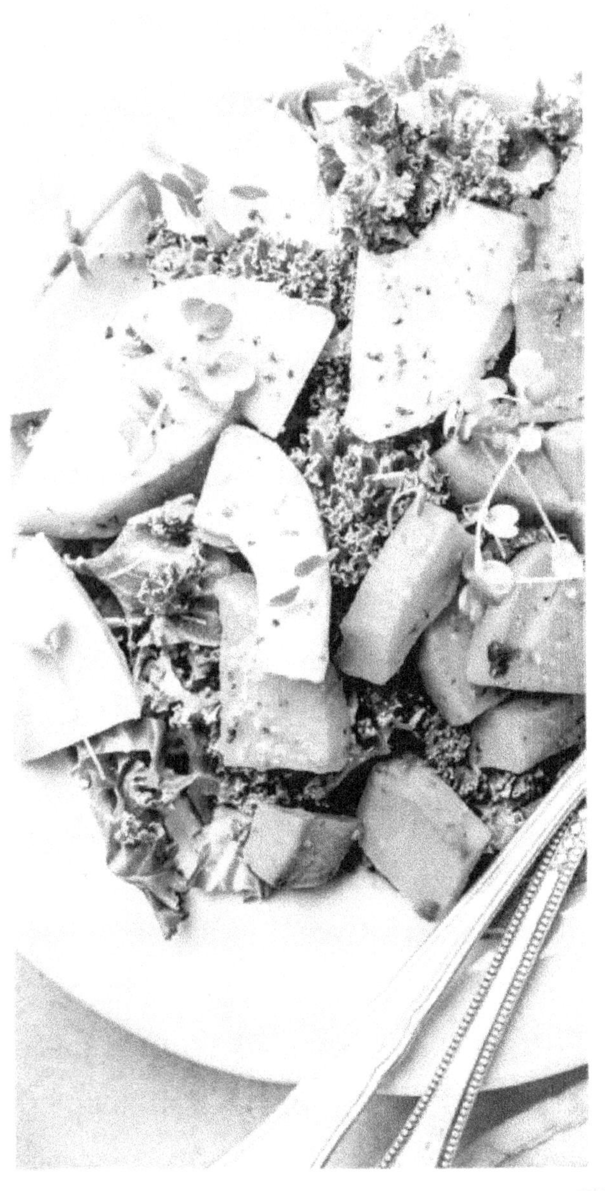

HOW CORTISOL DETOX AFFECTS WEIGHT LOSS AND HEALTH

A cortisol detox can significantly impact both weight loss and overall health by helping regulate the body's stress response and hormonal balance. When cortisol levels are consistently elevated due to chronic stress, it can hinder weight loss efforts and negatively affect physical and mental health. Detoxing cortisol—through proper nutrition, stress management, and lifestyle adjustments—helps rebalance hormone levels, which in turn aids weight management and improves well-being.

1. Reduction of Belly Fat and Weight Loss

One of the most notable effects of elevated cortisol is its tendency to increase fat storage, particularly in the abdominal area. High cortisol levels can trigger cravings for high-calorie, sugary foods and encourage fat storage in the body, contributing to weight gain and making it difficult to lose excess pounds. A cortisol detox aims to lower these levels, helping to reduce cravings, balance blood sugar levels, and enhance the body's ability to burn fat. This can lead to more effective weight loss, particularly around the belly, which is often the most stubborn area for fat reduction.

2. Balancing Blood Sugar and Reducing Insulin Resistance

Cortisol plays a role in regulating blood sugar by triggering the release of glucose into the bloodstream for quick energy. However, chronically high cortisol can lead to elevated blood sugar and eventually insulin resistance, a condition where cells become less responsive to insulin. This can impede weight loss and potentially lead to metabolic issues like type 2 diabetes. Detoxing cortisol helps stabilize blood sugar levels, reduces insulin spikes, and improves insulin sensitivity. This balanced state makes it easier for the body to utilize stored fat for energy and achieve sustainable weight loss.

3. Improved Metabolism and Appetite Regulation

Cortisol influences how the body metabolizes carbohydrates, fats, and proteins. When cortisol is too high, it can slow down the metabolism and promote muscle breakdown (catabolism), which reduces the body's ability to burn calories efficiently.

Detoxing cortisol helps reset and optimize metabolism, promoting muscle maintenance and improved fat burning. Additionally, regulating cortisol helps balance appetite-controlling hormones such as leptin (satiety hormone) and ghrelin (hunger hormone), aiding in better appetite control and reducing overeating.

4. Reduced Stress Eating and Emotional Eating

High cortisol levels often lead to emotional eating or "stress eating," where individuals crave comfort foods high in sugar and fat as a way to cope with stress. This pattern can hinder weight loss and lead to further weight gain. A cortisol detox encourages stress management techniques like meditation, regular exercise, and mindfulness practices, which help reduce the urge to eat in response to stress. By managing stress and lowering cortisol, emotional eating is minimized, making it easier to follow a balanced diet and adhere to weight loss goals.

5. Better Sleep and Recovery

Cortisol is linked to the body's sleep-wake cycle, and elevated levels, especially in the evening, can disrupt sleep patterns and reduce sleep quality. Poor sleep further raises cortisol levels and creates a cycle of stress and sleeplessness that negatively impacts weight loss efforts. A cortisol detox, which includes proper sleep hygiene, promotes better sleep quality and duration, allowing the body to recover, regulate hormones, and support weight loss more effectively.

6. Enhanced Muscle Mass and Physical Performance

Cortisol can break down muscle tissue for energy, particularly when levels are elevated due to stress. This muscle loss not only reduces strength but also lowers the

3. Improved Metabolism and Appetite Regulation

Cortisol influences how the body metabolizes carbohydrates, fats, and proteins. When cortisol is too high, it can slow down the metabolism and promote muscle breakdown (catabolism), which reduces the body's ability to burn calories efficiently.

Detoxing cortisol helps reset and optimize metabolism, promoting muscle maintenance and improved fat burning. Additionally, regulating cortisol helps balance appetite-controlling hormones such as leptin (satiety hormone) and ghrelin (hunger hormone), aiding in better appetite control and reducing overeating.

4. Reduced Stress Eating and Emotional Eating

High cortisol levels often lead to emotional eating or "stress eating," where individuals crave comfort foods high in sugar and fat as a way to cope with stress. This pattern can hinder weight loss and lead to further weight gain. A cortisol detox encourages stress management techniques like meditation, resting metabolic rate, making it harder to lose weight. A detox that focuses on balancing cortisol promotes muscle preservation, supporting lean muscle mass and improving overall physical performance. With more lean muscle, the body burns more calories at rest, aiding in weight loss and supporting overall physical health.

7. Improved Mental Health and Overall Well-being

By detoxing cortisol, mental health improves as anxiety, depression, and mood swings are reduced. A balanced cortisol level enhances focus, emotional stability, and resilience to stress, all of which are crucial for adhering to healthy lifestyle changes necessary for weight loss.

Improved mental health also supports more consistent exercise routines, healthier food choices, and better self-care, which are all beneficial to weight loss and overall health.

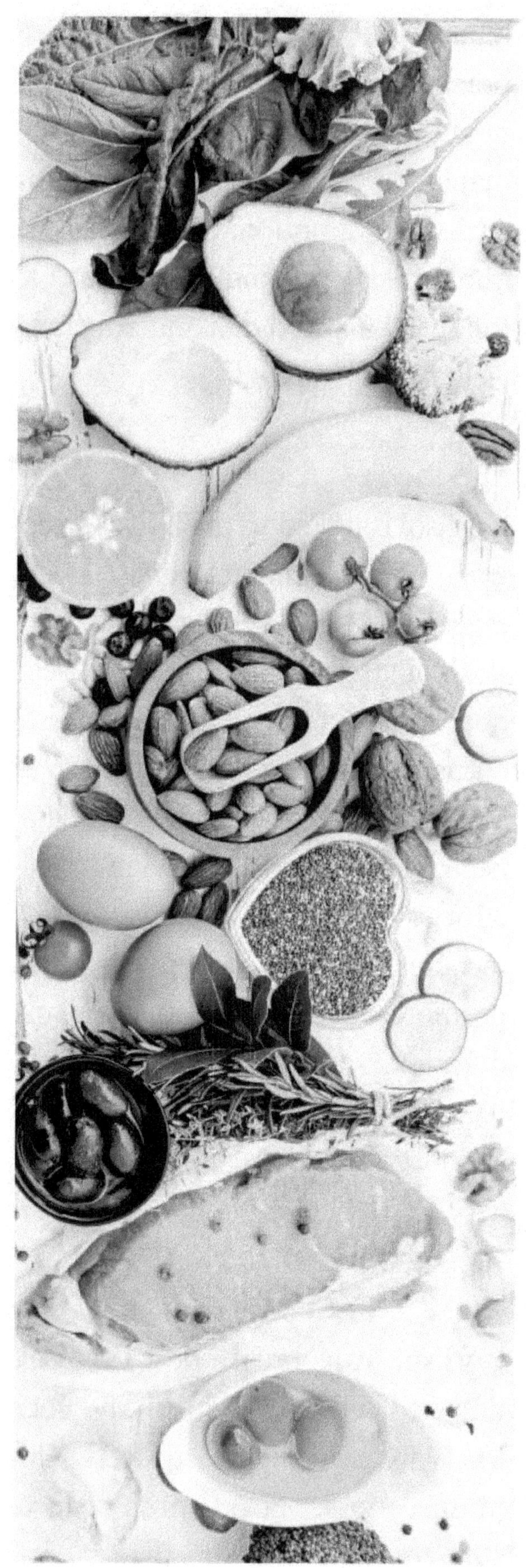

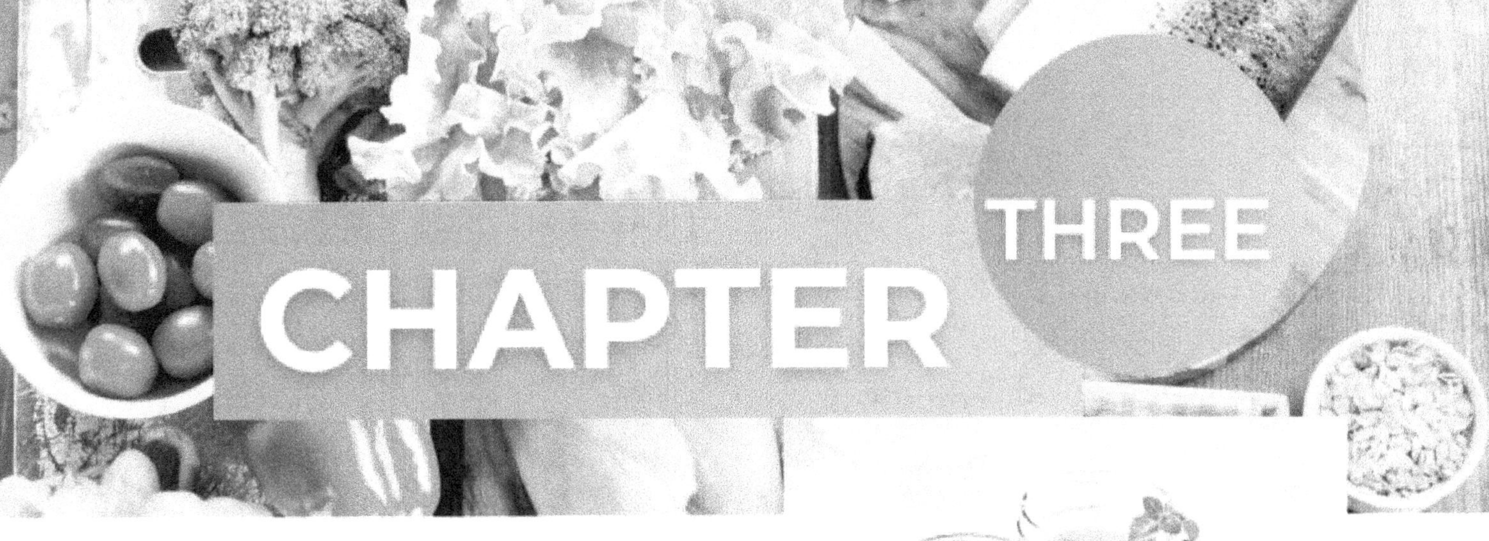

CHAPTER THREE

BENEFITS OF CORTISOL DETOX DIET

A Cortisol Detox Diet aims to help the body manage and regulate cortisol levels, ultimately improving physical and mental health. Below are the core benefits of following a Cortisol Detox Diet:

1. Reduced Stress and Anxiety

One of the primary benefits of a cortisol detox diet is its ability to reduce overall stress levels. The diet incorporates nutrient-dense foods that help stabilize blood sugar levels and promote the production of calming neurotransmitters like serotonin. This can lead to a more balanced emotional state, reduced anxiety, and an improved ability to cope with stress.

2. Improved Sleep Quality

Chronic stress and high cortisol disrupt the sleep-wake cycle, causing insomnia or poor-quality sleep. By consuming foods that support cortisol regulation, such as magnesium-rich leafy greens, nuts, and whole grains, the body can better manage its natural circadian rhythm. The result is more restful sleep, which contributes to better overall health and hormone balance.

3. Enhanced Weight Loss and Fat Reduction

High cortisol levels can promote fat storage, particularly around the abdominal area. A cortisol detox diet emphasizes balanced meals, with an adequate amount of protein, healthy fats, and fiber, to stabilize blood sugar and reduce cravings for sugary or processed foods.

This balanced approach supports the body's natural fat-burning process, making weight loss more effective and sustainable.

4. Stabilized Blood Sugar Levels

The diet focuses on consuming low glycemic index foods like whole grains, lean proteins, fruits, and vegetables, which helps regulate blood sugar levels. Consistent blood sugar regulation prevents the spikes and crashes that often trigger cortisol release, thus reducing the stress hormone's negative impact on the body.

This stabilization also helps prevent insulin resistance and supports better metabolic health.

5. Boosted Immune Function

Cortisol in excess can suppress the immune system, leading to increased susceptibility to infections and slower recovery. By focusing on anti-inflammatory foods like berries, citrus fruits, green tea, and fatty fish, the diet supports the body's natural defenses.

The inclusion of antioxidants, vitamins, and minerals strengthens the immune system and reduces inflammation, promoting overall health.

6. Enhanced Mental Clarity and Cognitive Function

Chronic stress and elevated cortisol levels can impair memory, concentration, and cognitive function.

The diet's focus on brain-supporting nutrients—such as omega-3 fatty acids, antioxidants, and B vitamins—enhances mental clarity, supports brain health, and may help improve memory and learning ability.

7. Balanced Hormones and Improved Mood

Cortisol is interconnected with other hormones, including insulin, estrogen, and testosterone. A cortisol detox diet helps balance these hormones by reducing stress and ensuring the body has adequate nutrients to produce and regulate them effectively.

A balanced hormonal system results in improved mood, better emotional regulation, and increased energy levels.

8. Reduced Inflammation and Pain Relief

Inflammation is closely tied to cortisol and stress. The diet's emphasis on anti-inflammatory foods—like turmeric, ginger, olive oil, and leafy greens—helps reduce inflammation in the body, leading to relief from chronic pain, joint issues, and other inflammatory conditions.

Reducing inflammation also supports cardiovascular health and reduces the risk of chronic diseases.

9. Improved Digestive Health

Chronic stress can negatively impact gut health, leading to digestive issues such as bloating, constipation, or irritable bowel syndrome (IBS).

A cortisol detox diet emphasizes gut-friendly foods such as fermented vegetables, yogurt, kefir, and high-fiber foods that support healthy digestion and promote a balanced gut microbiome.

A healthier gut enhances nutrient absorption and reduces gastrointestinal discomfort.

10. Better Energy Levels and Stamina

High cortisol can lead to adrenal fatigue, resulting in tiredness and low energy.

The diet helps regulate cortisol production and provides sustained energy through balanced macronutrients (proteins, fats, and complex carbs) and nutrient-rich foods.

This balance prevents energy crashes and promotes steady energy throughout the day, supporting better stamina and physical performance.

11. Enhanced Skin Health

Excess cortisol can affect the skin by promoting conditions like acne, eczema, or premature aging.

By detoxifying cortisol, the diet improves hormonal balance and reduces inflammation, leading to clearer and more radiant skin. Antioxidant-rich foods such as berries, citrus fruits, nuts, and seeds contribute to skin repair and overall skin health.

12. Supports Muscle Health and Prevents Muscle Loss

High cortisol can cause muscle breakdown (catabolism) as the body seeks to convert proteins into glucose for energy.

A cortisol detox diet, with its focus on lean proteins and muscle-supporting nutrients (like magnesium and B vitamins), helps maintain muscle mass and supports muscle repair and growth, enhancing physical health and strength.

FOODS TO AVOID AND INCLUDE

The Complete Cortisol Detox Diet Plan is designed to help balance cortisol levels through specific dietary choices that support stress management, hormonal balance, and overall well-being. By including certain foods and avoiding others, you can regulate cortisol production and optimize your physical and mental health.

Foods to Eat on a Cortisol Detox Diet

Whole Grains and Complex Carbohydrates

Complex carbohydrates like whole grains (brown rice, quinoa, oats, barley), legumes (lentils, chickpeas), and starchy vegetables (sweet potatoes, butternut squash) are essential for maintaining steady blood sugar levels, which is crucial for regulating cortisol. These foods provide sustained energy without causing spikes in blood sugar, which can trigger cortisol production.

Vegetables like spinach, kale, broccoli, and Brussels sprouts are rich in magnesium, a mineral that helps reduce stress and cortisol levels. Additionally, cruciferous vegetables (like cauliflower and broccoli) support liver detoxification, which helps eliminate excess cortisol from the body. A diverse range of colorful vegetables provides antioxidants that combat oxidative stress, a factor in elevated cortisol.

Healthy fats from sources like avocados, nuts (almonds, walnuts), seeds (chia, flax, pumpkin), olive oil, and fatty fish (salmon, mackerel, sardines) help stabilize blood sugar and provide anti-inflammatory benefits. Omega-3 fatty acids in fatty fish are particularly effective in reducing inflammation and regulating cortisol.

Including lean protein in your meals helps stabilize blood sugar levels and promotes satiety, both of which are essential for cortisol regulation. Good sources of lean protein include chicken, turkey, eggs, tofu, beans, lentils, and yogurt. Incorporating protein in every meal prevents hunger-induced stress and supports muscle health, which is often compromised by high cortisol.

Adaptogens like ashwagandha, rhodiola, and holy basil have natural properties that help the body adapt to stress and balance cortisol. Herbal teas such as chamomile, lavender, and green tea are calming and can lower cortisol levels, especially when consumed regularly as part of a relaxation routine.

Citrus fruits like oranges, lemons, grapefruits, and other vitamin C-rich fruits like strawberries, kiwi, and papaya support adrenal health and help reduce cortisol production. Vitamin C is a crucial nutrient for immune function and combating the effects of stress on the body.

Gut health is closely related to cortisol regulation. Including probiotic-rich foods like yogurt, kefir, sauerkraut, kimchi, and miso helps maintain a healthy gut microbiome, which in turn aids in hormone balance and stress response. A balanced gut helps reduce inflammation and supports better cortisol regulation.

Foods to Avoid on a Cortisol Detox Diet

Refined Sugars and Processed Carbohydrates

Foods high in refined sugars and simple carbs (white bread, pastries, sweets, sugary cereals) cause rapid spikes in blood sugar levels, leading to increased cortisol production. Consistently high blood sugar followed by crashes puts stress on the adrenal glands, disrupting cortisol balance and contributing to fatigue and weight gain.

Caffeine and Stimulants

Caffeine can elevate cortisol levels, especially when consumed in large quantities or late in the day. Coffee, energy drinks, and certain teas with high caffeine content can stimulate the adrenal glands and interfere with sleep patterns, further exacerbating cortisol production. While a moderate amount of caffeine may be tolerated, it is better to opt for green tea or herbal teas for their calming and cortisol-balancing effects.

Alcohol

Alcohol is a depressant that can increase cortisol production and disrupt sleep. Consuming alcohol regularly can lead to dehydration, poor sleep quality, and impaired stress response, all of which negatively affect cortisol levels. Reducing or eliminating alcohol consumption helps support the adrenal glands and cortisol detoxification.

High-Sodium and Processed Foods

Processed foods, often high in sodium and unhealthy fats (like trans fats and hydrogenated oils), can contribute to increased stress on the body and lead to water retention, hypertension, and inflammation.

Examples include fast food, chips, packaged snacks, and canned soups. These foods can negatively impact cortisol levels by disrupting the body's electrolyte balance and contributing to stress and anxiety.

Artificial Additives and Preservatives

Foods containing artificial additives, preservatives, and sweeteners (like aspartame or MSG) can trigger inflammatory responses and stress in the body, potentially leading to elevated cortisol levels. Reading labels and choosing whole, minimally processed foods is essential to avoid these hidden stressors.

Excessive Red Meat and High-Saturated Fat Foods

While lean proteins are encouraged, excessive consumption of red meat, fatty cuts of pork, and processed meats like bacon or sausage can increase inflammation and elevate cortisol levels. These foods are often high in saturated fats, which can contribute to cardiovascular stress and hormonal imbalance.

High Glycemic Index Fruits and Juices

Fruits with a high glycemic index (such as watermelon, pineapple, and overly ripe bananas) and fruit juices can quickly spike blood sugar levels, leading to increased cortisol production. It's better to consume whole fruits with lower glycemic indexes like berries, apples, and pears, which are also rich in fiber.

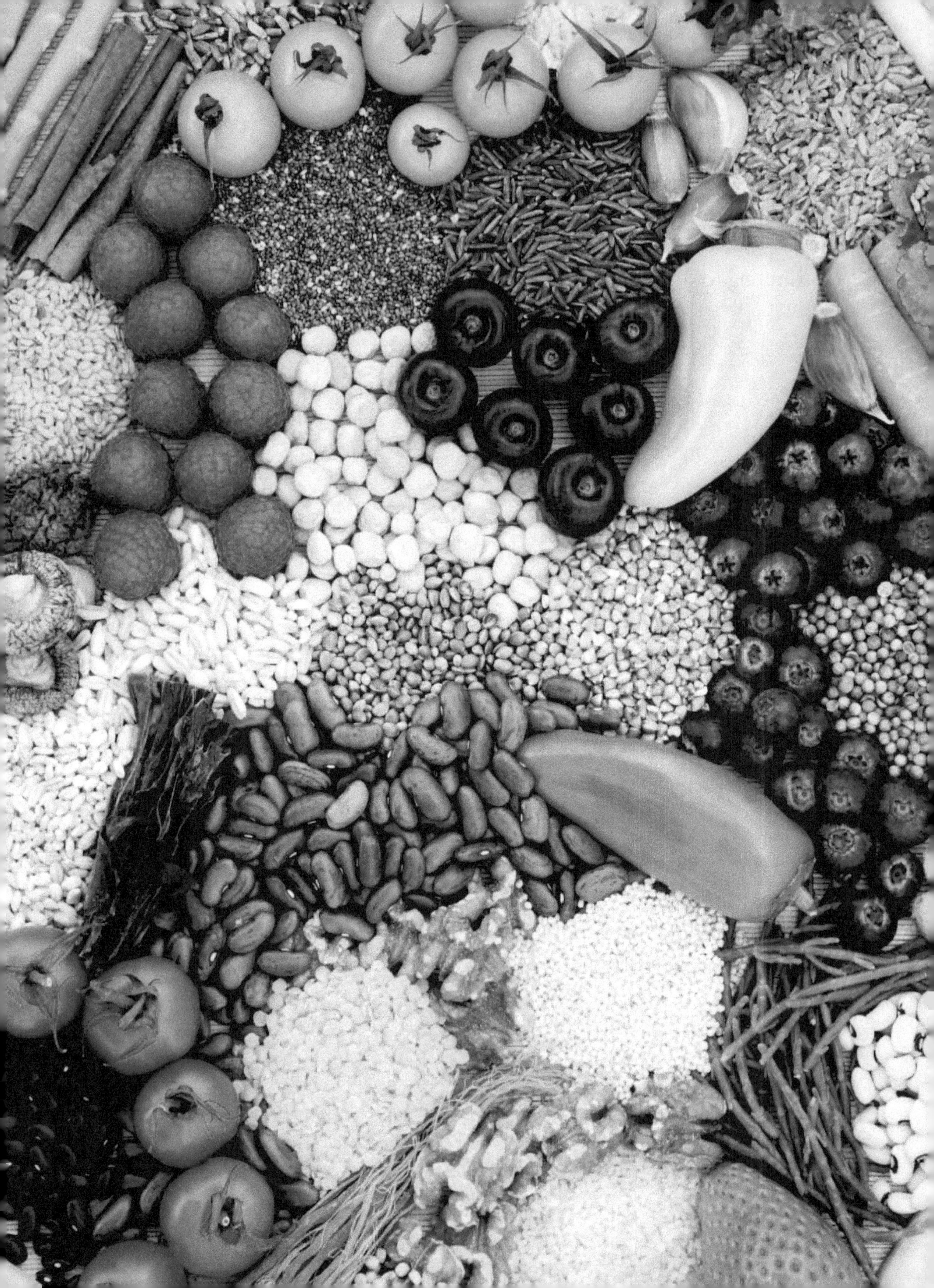

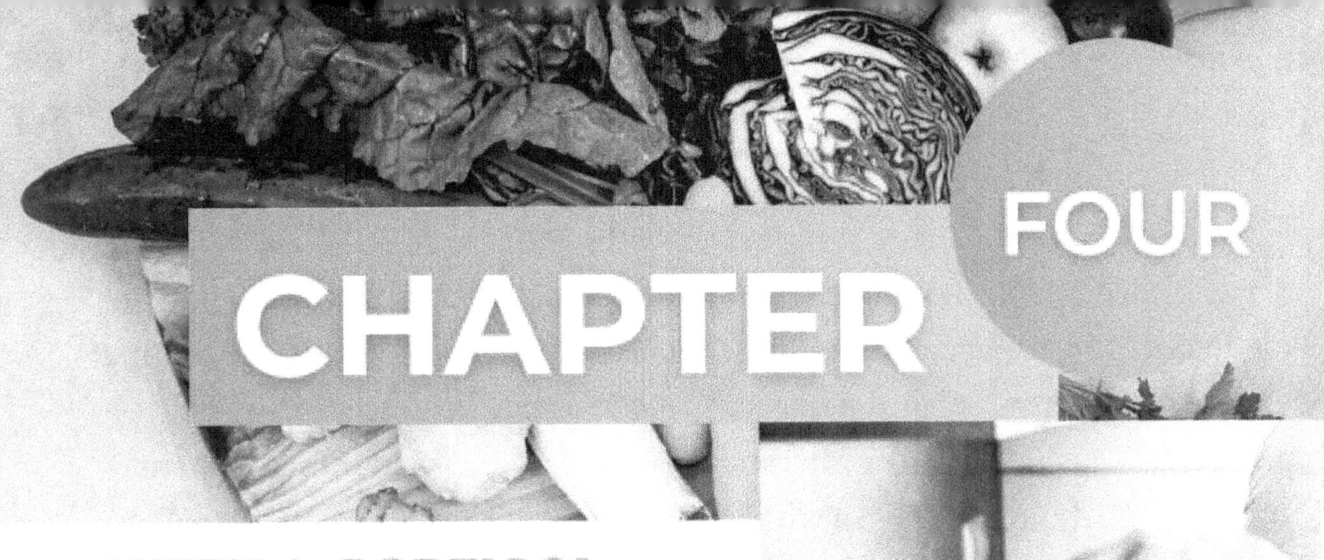

CHAPTER FOUR

WEEK 1: CORTISOL DETOX PREPARATION

Cortisol Detox Preparation involves readying your body and lifestyle to effectively reduce and balance cortisol levels. This preparation phase is crucial for setting the foundation for a successful cortisol detox and ensuring that the transition to a balanced, low-stress lifestyle is sustainable. Here's how to prepare for a cortisol detox:

1. Identify Stress Triggers and Lifestyle Factors

Begin by assessing the sources of stress in your life, which can be physical, emotional, or environmental. Recognize patterns of chronic stress, such as demanding work schedules, poor sleep habits, negative relationships, or unhealthy eating habits. By identifying these triggers, you can make a targeted plan to address them during the detox.

2. Create a Calming Environment

A cortisol detox is not just about food; it's also about creating a low-stress environment. Start by setting up a space at home dedicated to relaxation, free from distractions like electronic devices and work-related items. Incorporate calming elements like soothing lighting, aromatherapy (lavender or chamomile essential oils), and relaxing music to promote peace and help regulate cortisol.

3. Plan a Balanced, Anti-Inflammatory Diet

Proper nutrition plays a significant role in cortisol management. Before starting the detox, plan balanced meals that include lean proteins, complex carbohydrates, healthy fats, and a variety of fruits and vegetables. Make sure to shop for fresh, whole foods and avoid processed snacks, refined sugars, caffeine, and alcohol. Preparing meals in advance and keeping healthy snacks on hand can help you stick to the plan without feeling deprived.

4. Hydration and Herbal Teas

Ensure you're drinking plenty of water throughout the day, as proper hydration helps flush out toxins and maintain overall well-being. Including herbal teas like chamomile, peppermint, and green tea in your diet is beneficial for promoting relaxation and lowering cortisol. Try replacing caffeinated beverages with these herbal options to prepare your body for a caffeine reduction.

5. Establish a Consistent Sleep Routine

Sleep plays a significant role in cortisol regulation. Start by creating a consistent sleep routine where you go to bed and wake up at the same time every day, even on weekends. Aim for at least 7-9 hours of sleep each night. Preparing your sleep environment is also important—make sure your room is cool, dark, and free from electronic distractions, and establish a pre-bedtime routine that may include light stretching, reading, or meditation.

6. Incorporate Stress-Reduction Techniques

Start integrating stress-management practices into your daily routine before fully embarking on the detox. Techniques like meditation, deep breathing exercises, yoga, and progressive muscle relaxation help prepare the mind and body to manage stress more effectively and lower cortisol levels. Consistency is key, so find a method that works for you and make it a daily habit.

7. Gradually Reduce Caffeine and Alcohol Intake

High consumption of caffeine and alcohol can disrupt cortisol regulation and sleep patterns. Gradually reduce your intake of coffee, energy drinks, and alcohol before starting the detox to minimize withdrawal symptoms. Replace these beverages with herbal teas, water infused with lemon or cucumber, or other low-sugar, caffeine-free options.

8. Plan for Regular, Moderate Exercise

Physical activity helps regulate cortisol levels, but over-exercising can elevate cortisol due to physical stress. Prepare by planning moderate exercises such as walking, yoga, pilates, cycling, or light strength training.

Incorporate physical activity at least 3-5 times a week, ensuring it is enjoyable and not overly strenuous. Consistent, moderate exercise helps lower cortisol levels and promotes better mental and physical health.

9. Prepare Your Meals in Advance (Meal Prepping)

Meal prepping is an essential step in maintaining the cortisol detox diet. Plan and prepare meals and snacks for the week to avoid impulse eating or opting for less healthy options due to convenience. Focus on whole, nutrient-rich foods that support cortisol regulation, like lean proteins (chicken, fish, tofu), leafy greens, whole grains, nuts, and seeds. Keep fruits and vegetables washed, chopped, and ready to consume, and portion your meals to ensure balanced nutrition.

10. Practice Mindful Eating Habits

During a cortisol detox, it's not only what you eat but how you eat that matters. Begin to practice mindful eating by slowing down during meals, paying attention to flavors, and chewing food thoroughly. Avoid distractions like screens while eating, and make meals an opportunity to relax and enjoy your food. This mindful approach can help improve digestion, promote satiety, and reduce cortisol levels.

11. Manage Work and Life Balance

Evaluate your work-life balance and set boundaries to prevent burnout and chronic stress, which contribute to elevated cortisol. Establish clear work hours, delegate tasks when possible, and make time for hobbies, self-care, and family. Managing time effectively and allowing for relaxation helps keep cortisol levels in check.

12. Social Support and Accountability

A supportive network is key when preparing for a cortisol detox. Share your goals with family, friends, or a support group, and encourage them to help you stay accountable and motivated throughout the detox process. Having a community or accountability partner to discuss challenges and share progress can make the detox journey more effective and enjoyable.

Breakfast Recipes

Avocado and Spinach Toast

Ingredients

- 1 slice whole grain bread
- 1/2 ripe avocado
- Handful of spinach leaves
- A pinch of sea salt and black pepper
- Optional: a squeeze of lemon

Other Info

Nutrition (per serving):
- Calories: 200
- Healthy Fats: 14g
- Fiber: 6g
- Protein: 4g
- Servings: 1
- Cooking Time: 10 minutes

Directions

1. Toast the bread until golden.
2. Mash the avocado in a bowl and season with salt and pepper.
3. Sauté spinach in a pan until wilted.
4. Spread avocado on toast and top with sautéed spinach.
5. Optionally, squeeze a bit of lemon juice on top for flavor.
6. Serve immediately.

Blueberry Almond Overnight Oats

Ingredients

- 1/2 cup rolled oats
- 1/2 cup almond milk
- 1 tbsp almond butter
- 1/4 cup fresh blueberries
- A pinch of cinnamon

Other Info

Nutrition (per serving):
- Calories: 250
- Fiber: 7g
- Healthy Fats: 9g
- Protein: 6g
- Servings: 1
- Cooking Time: 5 minutes (plus overnight refrigeration)

Directions

1. In a jar, combine oats, almond milk, and almond butter.
2. Stir well to mix all ingredients.
3. Add blueberries on top and sprinkle with cinnamon.
4. Seal the jar and refrigerate overnight.
5. In the morning, stir and enjoy cold or warm it slightly.
6. Serve as is or topped with extra blueberries.

Greek Yogurt Parfait

Ingredients

- 1 cup Greek yogurt
- 1/2 cup mixed berries (strawberries, raspberries, blueberries)
- 1 tbsp chopped walnuts or almonds
- A drizzle of honey (optional)

Other Info

Nutrition (per serving):
- Calories: 200
- Protein: 14g
- Healthy Fats: 8g
- Fiber: 3g
- Servings: 1
- Cooking Time: 5 minutes

Directions

1. Layer half of the Greek yogurt in a glass or bowl.
2. Add a layer of mixed berries.
3. Top with the remaining yogurt.
4. Sprinkle with nuts and drizzle with honey if desired.
5. Enjoy immediately as a fresh, chilled breakfast.
6. Mix gently if preferred.

Banana and Chia Seed Smoothie

Ingredients

- 1 ripe banana
- 1 tbsp chia seeds
- 1 cup almond milk
- 1/2 tsp cinnamon
- A few ice cubes (optional)

Other Info

Nutrition (per serving):

- Calories: 180
- Fiber: 6g
- Healthy Fats: 5g
- Protein: 4g
- Servings: 1
- Cooking Time: 5 minutes

Directions

1. Peel and slice the banana.
2. In a blender, add banana, chia seeds, almond milk, and cinnamon.
3. Blend until smooth and creamy.
4. Add ice cubes if you prefer a chilled smoothie.
5. Pour into a glass and serve immediately.
6. Enjoy as a quick, refreshing breakfast.

Scrambled Eggs with Tomato and Basil

Ingredients

- 2 large eggs
- 1 small tomato, diced
- Fresh basil leaves, chopped
- 1 tsp olive oil
- A pinch of salt and pepper

Other Info

Nutrition (per serving):

- Calories: 160
- Protein: 12g
- Healthy Fats: 10g
- Fiber: 2g
- Servings: 1
- Cooking Time: 8 minutes

Directions

1. Whisk eggs in a bowl with a pinch of salt and pepper.
2. Heat olive oil in a non-stick pan over medium heat.
3. Add diced tomato and sauté for 1-2 minutes until softened.
4. Pour in the eggs and scramble gently until cooked.
5. Stir in fresh basil just before serving.
6. Serve hot with an optional side of whole-grain toast.

Lunch Recipes

Quinoa and Chickpea Salad

Ingredients

- 1/2 cup cooked quinoa
- 1/2 cup canned chickpeas (drained and rinsed)
- 1/2 cucumber, diced
- 1/4 cup cherry tomatoes, halved
- 1 tbsp olive oil and lemon juice for dressing
- A pinch of salt and pepper

Other Info

Nutrition (per serving):

- Calories: 250
- Protein: 9g
- Fiber: 7g
- Healthy Fats: 8g
- Servings: 1
- Cooking Time: 10 minutes (using pre-cooked quinoa)

Directions

1. In a bowl, combine quinoa, chickpeas, cucumber, and cherry tomatoes.
2. Drizzle olive oil and lemon juice over the salad.
3. Season with salt and pepper.
4. Mix thoroughly to coat everything with the dressing.
5. Let sit for 5 minutes for flavors to meld.
6. Serve chilled or at room temperature.

Turkey and Spinach Wrap

Ingredients

- 1 whole wheat tortilla
- 3 slices of turkey breast
- Handful of fresh spinach
- 1/4 avocado, sliced
- 1 tbsp hummus

Other Info

Nutrition (per serving):

- Calories: 280
- Protein: 15g
- Healthy Fats: 12g
- Fiber: 6g
- Servings: 1
- Cooking Time: 5 minutes

Directions

1. Lay the tortilla flat and spread hummus over it.
2. Add turkey slices, spinach, and avocado on top.
3. Roll the tortilla tightly into a wrap.
4. Cut in half for easy serving.
5. Serve with a side of mixed greens if desired.
6. Enjoy immediately or pack for a to-go lunch.

Lentil and Veggie Soup

Ingredients

- 1/2 cup cooked lentils
- 1 carrot, diced
- 1 celery stalk, chopped
- 1/2 onion, chopped
- 2 cups vegetable broth
- A pinch of salt and pepper

Other Info

Nutrition (per serving):

- Calories: 220
- Protein: 11g
- Fiber: 8g
- Healthy Fats: 2g
- Servings: 1
- Cooking Time: 15 minutes

Directions

1. In a pot, sauté onion, carrot, and celery until softened.
2. Add cooked lentils and vegetable broth.
3. Bring to a boil, then reduce heat and simmer for 10 minutes.
4. Season with salt and pepper.
5. Serve hot with a side of whole grain crackers if desired.
6. Enjoy a warming, nutritious lunch.

Grilled Chicken and Avocado Salad

Ingredients

- 1 grilled chicken breast (sliced)
- 1/2 avocado, diced
- Mixed greens (spinach, arugula, lettuce)
- 1 tbsp olive oil
- 1 tsp balsamic vinegar

Other Info

Nutrition (per serving):

- Calories: 300
- Protein: 20g
- Healthy Fats: 15g
- Fiber: 6g
- Servings: 1
- Cooking Time: 10 minutes (using pre-cooked chicken)

Directions

1. In a bowl, add mixed greens as a base.
2. Top with grilled chicken slices and avocado.
3. Drizzle olive oil and balsamic vinegar over the salad.
4. Toss gently to mix the dressing.
5. Season with salt and pepper if desired.
6. Serve fresh and enjoy.

Veggie and Brown Rice Stir-Fry

Ingredients

- 1/2 cup cooked brown rice
- 1/2 bell pepper, sliced
- 1/2 zucchini, diced
- 1 carrot, julienned
- 1 tbsp soy sauce
- 1 tsp olive oil

Other Info

Nutrition (per serving):

- Calories: 250
- Protein: 6g
- Fiber: 5g
- Healthy Fats: 4g
- Servings: 1
- Cooking Time: 10 minutes (using pre-cooked rice)

Directions

1. Heat olive oil in a pan over medium heat.
2. Add bell pepper, zucchini, and carrot, stir-frying for 3-4 minutes.
3. Stir in the cooked brown rice.
4. Add soy sauce and mix thoroughly.
5. Cook for another 2 minutes until heated through.
6. Serve warm as a balanced, colorful lunch.

Dinner Recipes

Baked Salmon with Asparagus

Ingredients

- 1 salmon fillet (about 4 oz)
- 1 cup asparagus spears
- 1 tbsp olive oil
- A pinch of salt and pepper
- Lemon wedge for serving

Other Info

Nutrition (per serving):

- Calories: 300
- Protein: 25g
- Healthy Fats: 18g
- Omega-3 Fatty Acids: High
- Servings: 1
- Cooking Time: 20 minutes

Directions

1. Preheat oven to 375°F (190°C).
2. Place salmon and asparagus on a baking tray; drizzle with olive oil.
3. Season with salt and pepper.
4. Bake for 15 minutes until salmon is cooked through and asparagus is tender.
5. Squeeze lemon juice over salmon before serving.
6. Serve hot with an optional side salad.

Quinoa and Veggie Stuffed Peppers

Ingredients

- 1 bell pepper (any color)
- 1/2 cup cooked quinoa
- 1/4 cup diced tomatoes
- 1/4 cup black beans (drained and rinsed)
- A pinch of cumin and salt

Other Info

Nutrition (per serving):

- Calories: 200
- Protein: 8g
- Fiber: 7g
- Healthy Fats: 3g
- Servings: 1
- Cooking Time: 30 minutes

Directions

1. Preheat oven to 375°F (190°C).
2. Mix quinoa, tomatoes, black beans, cumin, and salt in a bowl.
3. Cut the top off the bell pepper, remove seeds, and stuff with the quinoa mixture.
4. Place stuffed pepper in a baking dish and cover with foil.
5. Bake for 20-25 minutes until pepper is tender.
6. Serve warm.

Lemon-Garlic Shrimp and Broccoli

Ingredients

- 10-12 shrimp (peeled and deveined)
- 1 cup broccoli florets
- 1 tbsp olive oil
- 1 garlic clove, minced
- Juice of 1/2 lemon

Other Info

Nutrition (per serving):

- Calories: 220
- Protein: 20g
- Healthy Fats: 10g
- Fiber: 4g
- Servings: 1
- Cooking Time: 10 minutes

Directions

1. Heat olive oil in a pan over medium heat.
2. Add minced garlic and sauté for 1 minute.
3. Add shrimp and broccoli; cook for 3-4 minutes until shrimp turns pink.
4. Squeeze lemon juice over the shrimp and broccoli.
5. Stir for another minute until everything is well coated.
6. Serve immediately.

Sweet Potato and Lentil Curry

Ingredients

- 1/2 cup diced sweet potato
- 1/2 cup cooked lentils
- 1/4 cup coconut milk
- 1 tsp curry powder
- 1 tbsp olive oil

Other Info

Nutrition (per serving):

- Calories: 240
- Protein: 9g
- Fiber: 8g
- Healthy Fats: 8g
- Servings: 1
- Cooking Time: 15 minutes

Directions

1. Heat olive oil in a pan over medium heat.
2. Add diced sweet potato and sauté until slightly tender (about 5 minutes).
3. Stir in lentils and curry powder, mixing well.
4. Add coconut milk and simmer for 5 more minutes until sweet potato is fully tender.
5. Season with salt if needed.
6. Serve warm as a hearty dinner.

Zucchini Noodles with Pesto and Cherry Tomatoes

Ingredients

- 1 zucchini (spiralized into noodles)
- 1/4 cup cherry tomatoes, halved
- 1 tbsp pesto (store-bought or homemade)
- 1 tbsp olive oil
- A pinch of salt and pepper

Other Info

Nutrition (per serving):

- Calories: 180
- Healthy Fats: 12g
- Fiber: 4g
- Protein: 3g
- Servings: 1
- Cooking Time: 10 minutes

Directions

1. Heat olive oil in a pan over medium heat.
2. Add zucchini noodles and sauté for 2-3 minutes until slightly tender.
3. Stir in cherry tomatoes and cook for another minute.
4. Add pesto and toss to coat evenly.
5. Season with salt and pepper as desired.
6. Serve immediately as a light dinner option.

Snacks

Recipes

Apple Slices with Almond Butter

Ingredients

- 1 apple (sliced)
- 1 tbsp almond butter
- A pinch of cinnamon (optional)

Other Info

Nutrition (per serving):

- Calories: 150
- Fiber: 4g
- Healthy Fats: 8g
- Protein: 3g
- Servings: 1
- Cooking Time: 5 minutes

Directions

1. Core and slice the apple into thin wedges.
2. Spread almond butter on each apple slice.
3. Optionally, sprinkle cinnamon over the apple slices.
4. Arrange on a plate and enjoy as a quick snack.
5. Serve immediately to maintain freshness.
6. Pair with herbal tea if desired.

Greek Yogurt with Berries

Ingredients

- 1/2 cup Greek yogurt
- 1/4 cup mixed berries (blueberries, strawberries, raspberries)
- 1 tsp honey (optional)

Other Info

Nutrition (per serving):

- Calories: 120
- Protein: 10g
- Fiber: 3g
- Healthy Fats: 2g
- Servings: 1
- Cooking Time: 5 minutes

Directions

1. Scoop the Greek yogurt into a bowl.
2. Add mixed berries on top.
3. Drizzle honey over the berries if using.
4. Mix gently or leave as is for a layered effect.
5. Enjoy immediately as a refreshing snack.
6. Optionally, add a sprinkle of nuts or seeds for crunch.

Cucumber and Hummus Bites

Ingredients

- 1 cucumber (sliced into rounds)
- 2 tbsp hummus
- A pinch of paprika (optional)

Other Info

Nutrition (per serving):

- Calories: 80
- Fiber: 2g
- Healthy Fats: 4g
- Protein: 3g
- Servings: 1
- Cooking Time: 5 minutes

Directions

1. Slice the cucumber into 1/4-inch rounds.
2. Place a small dollop of hummus on each cucumber slice.
3. Optionally, sprinkle a pinch of paprika on top.
4. Arrange the bites on a plate.
5. Serve immediately as a light and crunchy snack.
6. Enjoy with herbal tea or water.

Carrot and Avocado Dip

Ingredients

- 1 carrot (cut into sticks)
- 1/4 ripe avocado
- A squeeze of lemon juice
- A pinch of salt and pepper

Other Info

Nutrition (per serving):

- Calories: 100
- Fiber: 5g
- Healthy Fats: 7g
- Protein: 1g
- Servings: 1
- Cooking Time: 5 minutes

Directions

1. Mash the avocado with lemon juice, salt, and pepper in a small bowl.
2. Cut the carrot into sticks for dipping.
3. Serve carrot sticks with the avocado dip on the side.
4. Enjoy as a fresh and crunchy snack.
5. Optionally, add other vegetable sticks like celery or cucumber.
6. Consume immediately to maintain freshness.

Almond and Dark Chocolate Mix

Ingredients

- 10 almonds
- 2 small squares of dark chocolate (70% cocoa or higher)

Other Info

Nutrition (per serving):

- Calories: 140
- Healthy Fats: 10g
- Protein: 3g
- Fiber: 3g
- Servings: 1
- Cooking Time: 2 minutes

Directions

1. Place almonds and dark chocolate on a small plate.
2. Break chocolate into smaller pieces if preferred.
3. Mix almonds and chocolate together.
4. Enjoy as a simple, satisfying snack.
5. Consume with a glass of water or herbal tea.
6. Store remaining almonds in an airtight container for future snacks.

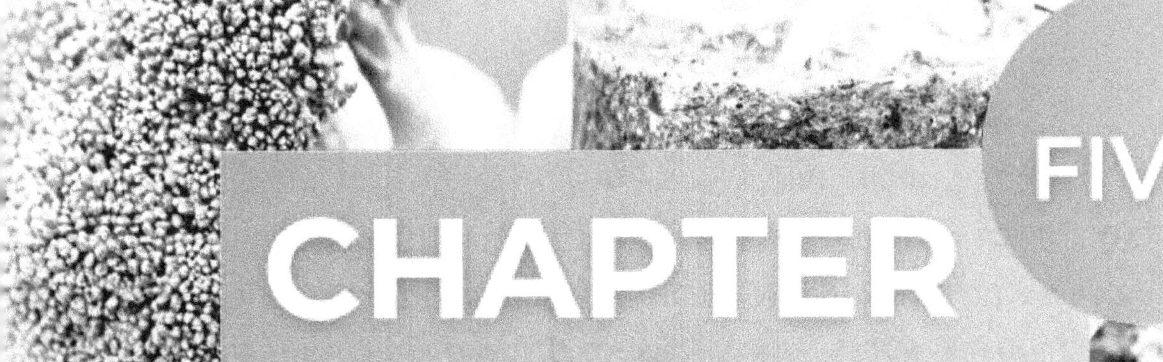

WEEK 2: HOW TO REDUCE CORTISOL LEVELS NATURALLY

Reducing cortisol levels naturally can significantly improve your overall well-being, stress management, and health. Here are several effective strategies to naturally lower cortisol:

1. Get Enough Sleep

Quality sleep is essential for regulating cortisol levels. Aim for 7-9 hours of restful sleep per night.

Establish a regular sleep schedule by going to bed and waking up at the same time each day.

Practice a relaxing bedtime routine (like reading or warm baths) to improve sleep quality.

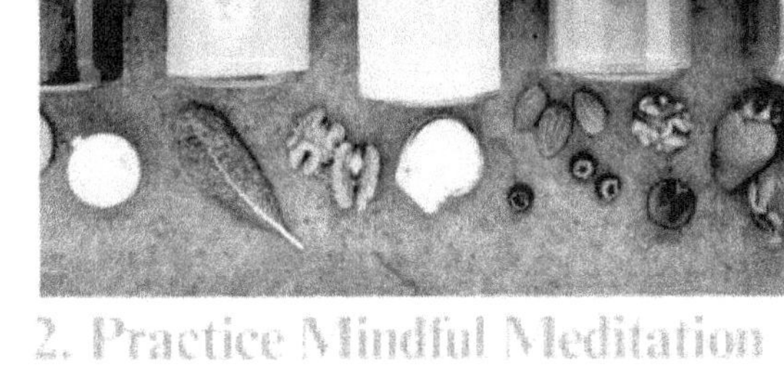

2. Practice Mindful Meditation and Relaxation

Meditation, deep breathing exercises, yoga, and progressive muscle relaxation can significantly lower stress and reduce cortisol levels.

Spend 5-10 minutes daily practicing mindfulness to focus on the present moment and calm your mind.

3. Maintain a Balanced Diet

Complex carbohydrates, such as whole grains, and foods rich in fiber and protein, help stabilize blood sugar levels and prevent cortisol spikes.

Include antioxidant-rich foods (e.g., berries, leafy greens, nuts) and omega-3 fatty acids (found in salmon, walnuts, chia seeds) to combat inflammation and stress.
Avoid refined sugars, processed foods, and excessive caffeine, which can contribute to elevated cortisol.

4. Stay Physically Active

Regular exercise helps reduce stress and lower cortisol levels, but moderation is key.
Opt for moderate-intensity exercises like walking, swimming, yoga, or cycling rather than high-intensity workouts, which can increase cortisol if done excessively.
Aim for 30 minutes of moderate activity most days of the week.

5. Stay Hydrated

Dehydration can trigger increased cortisol production.
Drink plenty of water throughout the day and include hydrating foods like fruits and vegetables in your diet.

6. Limit Stimulants (Caffeine and Alcohol)

High caffeine intake can stimulate cortisol production, especially when consumed in large amounts or late in the day.
Reduce or switch to herbal teas like chamomile, peppermint, or green tea, which promote relaxation.
Alcohol can also interfere with sleep and hormone regulation, so consider reducing your consumption.

7. Connect with Others

Positive social interactions can lower cortisol.
Spend time with friends, family, or pets, engage in enjoyable hobbies, and create meaningful connections to boost your mood and reduce stress.

8. Laugh and Have Fun

Laughter has been shown to reduce cortisol and improve mood.
Engage in activities that make you smile, such as watching a comedy, playing games, or spending time with loved ones.

9. Use Adaptogenic Herbs

Certain herbs, known as adaptogens, help the body manage stress and balance cortisol levels.
Ashwagandha, rhodiola, holy basil, and ginseng are examples of adaptogens that can support a healthy stress response.

10. Manage Time and Set Boundaries

Overworking or lack of work-life balance can contribute to high stress and cortisol levels.
Plan and organize your tasks, delegate when possible, and set clear boundaries to avoid burnout.

11. Incorporate Relaxing Activities

Activities like listening to music, taking nature walks, practicing aromatherapy (using lavender or chamomile essential oils), or engaging in a hobby can reduce cortisol and promote relaxation.

12. Practice Gratitude and Positive Thinking

Gratitude journaling and focusing on positive thoughts can shift your mindset and lower stress.
Start or end your day by writing down a few things you're thankful for to cultivate a positive outlook and reduce cortisol.

13. Balance Blood Sugar Levels

Consistent, balanced meals containing protein, healthy fats, and fiber can help keep blood sugar steady and prevent cortisol spikes.
Avoid skipping meals and eat regularly throughout the day.

By combining these natural methods, you can effectively reduce cortisol levels, improve your ability to manage stress, and enhance your overall physical and mental health.

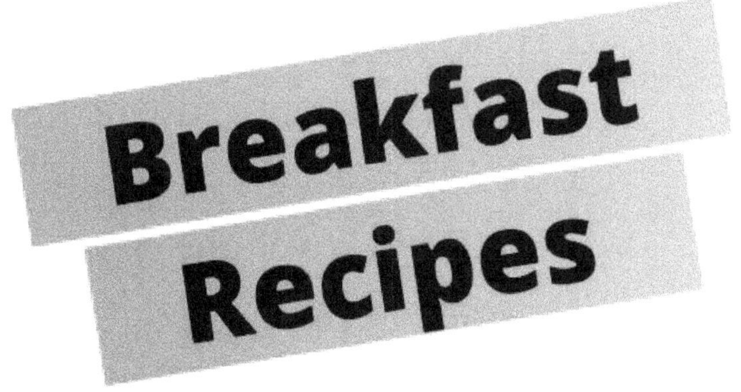

Spinach and Mushroom Omelette

Ingredients

- 2 eggs
- Handful of spinach
- 3-4 mushrooms, sliced
- 1 tsp olive oil
- Salt and pepper to taste

Other Info

Nutrition (per serving):

- Calories: 180
- Protein: 12g
- Healthy Fats: 11g
- Fiber: 2g
- Servings: 1
- Cooking Time: 10 minutes

Directions

1. Whisk eggs with salt and pepper in a bowl.
2. Heat olive oil in a pan over medium heat and sauté mushrooms until softened.
3. Add spinach and cook until wilted.
4. Pour eggs over the veggies and cook until set, folding the omelette in half.
5. Cook for another 1-2 minutes until done.
6. Serve warm with an optional side of whole grain toast.

Berry and Nut Chia Pudding

Ingredients

- 3 tbsp chia seeds
- 1 cup almond milk
- 1/4 cup mixed berries (blueberries, raspberries)
- 1 tbsp chopped almonds or walnuts

Other Info

Nutrition (per serving):

- Calories: 220
- Protein: 8g
- Healthy Fats: 10g
- Fiber: 11g
- Servings: 1
- Cooking Time: 5 minutes (plus refrigeration time)

Directions

1. In a jar, mix chia seeds and almond milk thoroughly.
2. Cover and refrigerate overnight or at least for 2 hours to thicken.
3. Before serving, top with mixed berries and nuts.
4. Stir gently and serve chilled.
5. Add more almond milk if needed for consistency.
6. Enjoy as a refreshing breakfast option.

Banana Oat Pancakes

Ingredients

- 1 ripe banana
- 1/2 cup rolled oats
- 1 egg
- 1/2 tsp cinnamon
- 1 tsp coconut oil (for cooking)

Other Info

Nutrition (per serving):

- Calories: 230
- Protein: 7g
- Healthy Fats: 6g
- Fiber: 5g
- Servings: 1
- Cooking Time: 10 minutes

Directions

1. Mash the banana in a bowl and mix in oats, egg, and cinnamon.
2. Heat coconut oil in a non-stick pan over medium heat.
3. Pour batter into small pancakes and cook for 2-3 minutes on each side until golden.
4. Flip carefully and cook through.
5. Serve warm with optional toppings like berries or a drizzle of honey.
6. Enjoy a nutritious start to your day.

Sweet Potato Breakfast Hash

Ingredients

- 1/2 cup diced sweet potato
- 1/4 bell pepper, diced
- 1/4 onion, diced
- 1 tbsp olive oil
- Salt and pepper to taste

Other Info

Nutrition (per serving):

- Calories: 180
- Fiber: 4g
- Healthy Fats: 7g
- Vitamin A: High
- Servings: 1
- Cooking Time: 15 minutes

Directions

1. Heat olive oil in a skillet over medium heat.
2. Add sweet potato and sauté for 5 minutes until slightly softened.
3. Stir in bell pepper and onion; cook until veggies are tender and slightly browned.
4. Season with salt and pepper.
5. Serve warm as is or with a side of scrambled eggs.
6. Enjoy a balanced, hearty breakfast.

Pear and Walnut Parfait

Ingredients

- 1 pear, diced
- 1/2 cup Greek yogurt
- 1 tbsp walnuts, chopped
- A sprinkle of ground flaxseed (optional)

Other Info

Nutrition (per serving):

- Calories: 200
- Protein: 10g
- Healthy Fats: 7g
- Fiber: 4g
- Servings: 1
- Cooking Time: 5 minutes

Directions

1. Spoon half the Greek yogurt into a bowl or glass.
2. Add half of the diced pear as a layer.
3. Repeat with the remaining yogurt and pear.
4. Top with chopped walnuts and flaxseed.
5. Enjoy immediately as a creamy, crunchy breakfast.
6. Optionally, drizzle with a little honey for sweetness.

Lunch Recipes

Mediterranean Chickpea Bowl

Ingredients

- 1/2 cup canned chickpeas (drained and rinsed)
- 1/4 cucumber, diced
- 1/4 cup cherry tomatoes, halved
- 1 tbsp olives, sliced
- 1 tbsp olive oil and lemon juice dressing

Other Info

Nutrition (per serving):

- Calories: 250
- Protein: 8g
- Fiber: 7g
- Healthy Fats: 10g
- Servings: 1
- Cooking Time: 10 minutes

Directions

1. In a bowl, mix chickpeas, cucumber, tomatoes, and olives.
2. Drizzle with olive oil and lemon juice.
3. Stir well to coat all ingredients evenly.
4. Let sit for 5 minutes for flavors to meld.
5. Season with salt and pepper as desired.
6. Serve fresh with an optional side of greens.

Lentil and Avocado Lettuce Wraps

Ingredients

- 1/2 cup cooked lentils
- 1/2 avocado, diced
- 2-3 large lettuce leaves
- A pinch of salt, pepper, and cumin for seasoning
- Optional: a squeeze of lime juice

Other Info

Nutrition (per serving):

- Calories: 200
- Protein: 8g
- Fiber: 8g
- Healthy Fats: 9g
- Servings: 1
- Cooking Time: 10 minutes

Directions

1. Mix cooked lentils and diced avocado in a bowl.
2. Season with salt, pepper, cumin, and lime juice if desired.
3. Lay lettuce leaves on a plate.
4. Spoon lentil and avocado mixture into each leaf.
5. Wrap leaves around the filling to create wraps.
6. Serve immediately for a light, refreshing lunch.

Brown Rice and Black Bean Bowl

Ingredients

- 1/2 cup cooked brown rice
- 1/4 cup canned black beans (drained and rinsed)
- 1/4 cup bell pepper, diced
- 1 tbsp salsa (mild or medium)
- A pinch of cumin and salt

Other Info

Nutrition (per serving):

- Calories: 230
- Protein: 8g
- Fiber: 6g
- Healthy Fats: 2g
- Servings: 1
- Cooking Time: 10 minutes

Directions

1. In a bowl, combine cooked brown rice, black beans, and bell pepper.
2. Add salsa and season with cumin and salt.
3. Stir well to mix all ingredients thoroughly.
4. Let sit for 2-3 minutes for flavors to combine.
5. Serve warm or at room temperature.
6. Garnish with cilantro if desired.

Tuna and Spinach Salad

Ingredients

- 1 can tuna in water (drained)
- 1 cup fresh spinach leaves
- 1/4 cucumber, sliced
- 1 tbsp olive oil
- 1 tsp balsamic vinegar

Other Info

Nutrition (per serving):

- Calories: 180
- Protein: 22g
- Healthy Fats: 9g
- Fiber: 2g
- Servings: 1
- Cooking Time: 5 minutes

Directions

1. Place spinach and cucumber in a bowl.
2. Add drained tuna on top.
3. Drizzle olive oil and balsamic vinegar over the salad.
4. Toss gently to coat all ingredients evenly.
5. Season with salt and pepper as desired.
6. Serve immediately.

Sweet Potato and Kale Sauté

Ingredients

- 1 small sweet potato (peeled and diced)
- 1 cup chopped kale
- 1 tbsp olive oil
- 1 garlic clove, minced
- A pinch of salt and pepper

Other Info

Nutrition (per serving):

- Calories: 200
- Fiber: 6g
- Healthy Fats: 7g
- Vitamin A: High
- Servings: 1
- Cooking Time: 15 minutes

Directions

1. Heat olive oil in a pan over medium heat.
2. Add sweet potato and sauté for 8-10 minutes until tender.
3. Add minced garlic and chopped kale to the pan.
4. Sauté for another 3-4 minutes until kale is wilted.
5. Season with salt and pepper to taste.
6. Serve warm as a nourishing, filling lunch.

Dinner Recipes

Grilled Lemon Herb Chicken with Zucchini

Ingredients

- 1 chicken breast (about 4 oz)
- 1 small zucchini, sliced
- Juice of 1/2 lemon
- 1 tbsp olive oil
- Salt, pepper, and dried herbs (thyme or oregano)

Other Info

Nutrition (per serving):

- Calories: 250
- Protein: 24g
- Healthy Fats: 12g
- Vitamin C: High
- Servings: 1
- Cooking Time: 15 minutes (plus marinating)

Directions

1. Marinate chicken in lemon juice, olive oil, salt, pepper, and herbs for 10 minutes.
2. Heat a grill pan over medium heat and grill chicken for 5-6 minutes on each side until cooked through.
3. Remove chicken and grill zucchini slices for 2 minutes per side.
4. Season zucchini with a pinch of salt and pepper.
5. Serve grilled chicken with zucchini on the side.
6. Optionally, garnish with lemon wedges.

Shrimp and Cauliflower Rice Stir-Fry

Ingredients

- 10 shrimp (peeled and deveined)
- 1 cup cauliflower rice
- 1/2 bell pepper, diced
- 1 tbsp soy sauce or tamari
- 1 tsp olive oil

Other Info

Nutrition (per serving):

- Calories: 220
- Protein: 22g
- Healthy Fats: 5g
- Fiber: 4g
- Servings: 1
- Cooking Time: 10 minutes

Directions

1. Heat olive oil in a pan over medium heat.
2. Add shrimp and cook until pink (about 3 minutes).
3. Remove shrimp and add bell pepper to the pan; sauté for 2 minutes.
4. Stir in cauliflower rice and soy sauce, cooking for 3 minutes until tender.
5. Add shrimp back to the pan and mix well.
6. Serve warm as a light, flavorful dinner.

Baked Cod with Cherry Tomatoes and Basil

Ingredients

- 1 cod fillet (about 4 oz)
- 1/2 cup cherry tomatoes, halved
- 1 tbsp olive oil
- Fresh basil leaves, chopped
- Salt and pepper to taste

Other Info

Nutrition (per serving):

- Calories: 180
- Protein: 24g
- Healthy Fats: 8g
- Omega-3 Fatty Acids: High
- Servings: 1
- Cooking Time: 20 minutes

Directions

1. Preheat oven to 375°F (190°C).
2. Place cod fillet and cherry tomatoes on a baking dish.
3. Drizzle with olive oil and season with salt and pepper.
4. Bake for 12-15 minutes until the fish is flaky and cooked through.
5. Garnish with fresh basil before serving.
6. Serve immediately.

Turkey and Veggie Skewers

Ingredients

- 4 oz turkey breast, cubed
- 1/2 bell pepper, cut into chunks
- 1/2 zucchini, sliced
- 1 tbsp olive oil
- Salt, pepper, and dried herbs (oregano or thyme)

Other Info

Nutrition (per serving):

- Calories: 200
- Protein: 25g
- Healthy Fats: 7g
- Fiber: 3g
- Servings: 1
- Cooking Time: 15 minutes

Directions

1. Preheat grill or grill pan over medium heat.
2. Thread turkey, bell pepper, and zucchini onto skewers.
3. Brush skewers with olive oil and season with salt, pepper, and herbs.
4. Grill for 8-10 minutes, turning occasionally, until turkey is cooked through.
5. Serve hot as a fun, nutritious dinner.
6. Pair with a side salad if desired.

Veggie and Tofu Stir-Fry

Ingredients

- 1/2 cup firm tofu, cubed
- 1/2 cup broccoli florets
- 1/2 carrot, julienned
- 1 tbsp soy sauce or tamari
- 1 tsp sesame oil

Other Info

Nutrition (per serving):

- Calories: 180
- Protein: 10g
- Healthy Fats: 8g
- Fiber: 4g
- Servings: 1
- Cooking Time: 10 minutes

Directions

1. Heat sesame oil in a pan over medium heat.
2. Add tofu cubes and sauté until golden (about 5 minutes).
3. Add broccoli and carrots, cooking for 3 minutes until slightly tender.
4. Stir in soy sauce and mix well.
5. Cook for another 2 minutes until flavors blend.
6. Serve warm with an optional sprinkle of sesame seeds.

Snacks

Recipes

Celery Sticks with Guacamole

Ingredients

- 2 celery stalks, cut into sticks
- 1/2 avocado, mashed
- Juice of 1/2 lime
- A pinch of salt and pepper

Other Info

Nutrition (per serving):

- Calories: 100
- Healthy Fats: 7g
- Fiber: 4g
- Vitamin C: High
- Servings: 1
- Cooking Time: 5 minutes

Directions

1. In a small bowl, mash the avocado and mix in lime juice, salt, and pepper.
2. Serve guacamole as a dip with celery sticks on the side.
3. Enjoy a crunchy, refreshing snack.
4. Add chopped tomatoes to guacamole for more flavor if desired.
5. Consume immediately for the best taste and texture.
6. Pack for on-the-go in a small container.

Almond Date Energy Bites

Ingredients

- 5 almonds
- 2 dates (pitted)
- 1/4 tsp cinnamon

Other Info

Nutrition (per serving):

- Calories: 120
- Healthy Fats: 6g
- Fiber: 3g
- Natural Sugars: Moderate
- Servings: 1 (makes about 2 bites)
- Cooking Time: 5 minutes (plus chilling)

Directions

1. Finely chop the almonds and dates.
2. Mix chopped almonds, dates, and cinnamon in a bowl until combined.
3. Roll mixture into small bite-sized balls.
4. Refrigerate for 10-15 minutes to set.
5. Serve as a quick energy-boosting snack.
6. Store extras in an airtight container.

Carrot and Apple Slices with Nut Butter

Ingredients

- 1 small carrot, cut into sticks
- 1/2 apple, sliced
- 1 tbsp cashew or almond butter

Other Info

Nutrition (per serving):

- Calories: 130
- Healthy Fats: 8g
- Fiber: 5g
- Natural Sugars: Low
- Servings: 1
- Cooking Time: 5 minutes

Directions

1. Arrange carrot sticks and apple slices on a plate.
2. Serve with a side of nut butter for dipping.
3. Optionally, sprinkle a pinch of cinnamon on apple slices for flavor.
4. Enjoy as a sweet and savory snack.
5. Keep fresh by storing apple slices in a bit of lemon water if preparing ahead.
6. Perfect for an afternoon pick-me-up.

Cucumber Mint Smoothie

Ingredients

- 1/2 cucumber, chopped
- A handful of fresh mint leaves
- 1/2 cup coconut water
- A squeeze of lime juice

Other Info

Nutrition (per serving):

- Calories: 40
- Fiber: 2g
- Hydration: High
- Natural Sugars: Very Low
- Servings: 1
- Cooking Time: 5 minutes

Directions

1. Add cucumber, mint, coconut water, and lime juice to a blender.
2. Blend until smooth.
3. Pour into a glass and serve immediately.
4. Optionally, add ice cubes for a chilled drink.
5. Garnish with extra mint leaves if desired.
6. Sip slowly and enjoy as a refreshing snack.

Roasted Pumpkin Seeds

Ingredients

- 1/4 cup raw pumpkin seeds
- 1 tsp olive oil
- A pinch of salt and paprika

Other Info

Nutrition (per serving):

- Calories: 90
- Healthy Fats: 7g
- Fiber: 2g
- Protein: 4g
- Servings: 1
- Cooking Time: 15 minutes

Directions

1. Preheat oven to 350°F (175°C).
2. Mix pumpkin seeds with olive oil, salt, and paprika.
3. Spread seeds on a baking sheet.
4. Roast for 10-12 minutes until golden brown, stirring halfway through.
5. Let cool before eating for a crunchy snack.
6. Store extras in an airtight container.

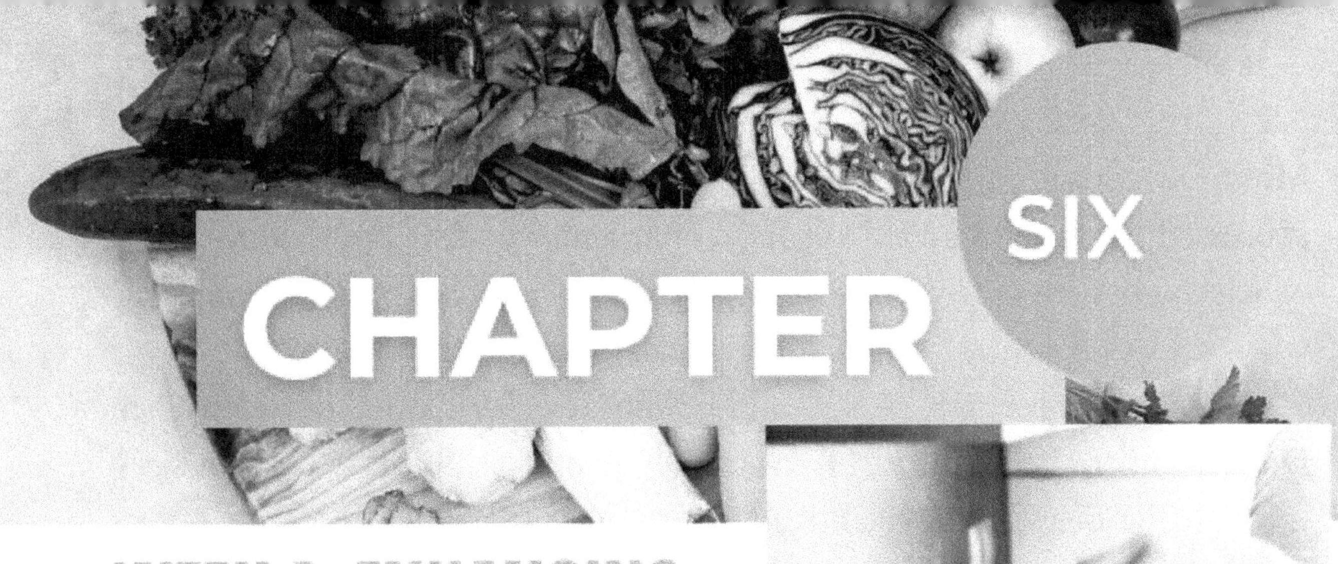

WEEK 3: ENHANCING DETOXIFICATION

Enhancing detoxification involves supporting your body's natural ability to eliminate toxins effectively. The body naturally detoxifies through the liver, kidneys, lungs, skin, and digestive system, and enhancing these processes can improve overall health and well-being. Here are several ways to enhance detoxification naturally:

1. Hydrate Adequately

Drinking plenty of water helps flush toxins out of your body, primarily through your kidneys and urine.

Aim for at least 8-10 glasses of water daily and include hydrating foods like cucumbers, watermelon, and leafy greens.

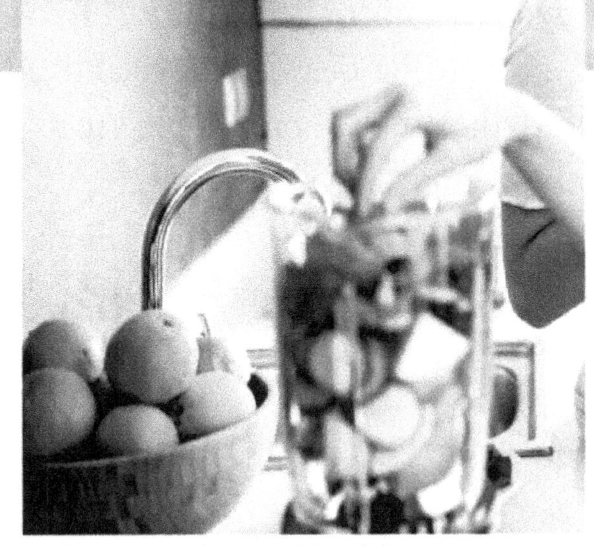

2. Support Liver Health

The liver is the main detoxification organ, and certain foods can support its function:

Cruciferous vegetables like broccoli, Brussels sprouts, cauliflower, and kale contain compounds that support liver detoxification enzymes.

Citrus fruits like lemons, oranges, and grapefruit are high in antioxidants and vitamin C, which help the liver cleanse the blood.

Beets, garlic, and turmeric are also known to enhance liver detox pathways.

Minimize consumption of alcohol, processed foods, and added sugars, which can burden the liver.

3. Eat Fiber-Rich Foods

Dietary fiber helps move toxins through the digestive tract and out of the body, promoting regular bowel movements.

Include whole grains, legumes, fruits, vegetables, nuts, and seeds in your diet to ensure adequate fiber intake.

Probiotic-rich foods like yogurt, kefir, sauerkraut, kimchi, and kombucha can improve gut health and support digestion, which enhances detoxification.

4. Sweat It Out

Sweating is a natural way the body eliminates toxins through the skin.

Engage in moderate exercises like jogging, cycling, or yoga to promote sweat production.

Saunas or steam baths are also effective ways to sweat and enhance detoxification.

5. Get Enough Sleep

Quality sleep allows the body to rest, repair, and detoxify itself, particularly the brain through a process known as glymphatic clearance.

Aim for 7-9 hours of sleep each night and establish a regular sleep routine to enhance the body's natural detoxification processes.

6. Support Lymphatic Drainage

The lymphatic system is responsible for carrying toxins away from tissues and into the bloodstream for elimination.

Gentle exercises like walking, swimming, and rebounding (using a mini trampoline) can promote lymphatic circulation.

Dry brushing the skin before a shower can stimulate lymph flow and improve detoxification through the skin.

7. Consume Antioxidant-Rich Foods

Antioxidants neutralize free radicals and help the body combat the damage caused by toxins.

Include berries, green tea, nuts, seeds, dark leafy greens, and spices like turmeric and ginger in your diet to support antioxidant activity.

Reducing exposure to environmental toxins, such as chemicals found in household cleaners, personal care products, plastics, and pollution, can decrease the toxic load on the body.

Opt for natural, non-toxic cleaning products, BPA-free containers, and organic or minimally processed foods when possible.

Deep breathing exercises help improve oxygen flow, which can enhance lung detoxification and promote better circulation.

Try 5-10 minutes of deep breathing exercises daily, focusing on slow, deep inhales and exhales to help eliminate toxins through the lungs.

Chronic inflammation can hinder detoxification pathways.

Include anti-inflammatory foods like omega-3 fatty acids (from fatty fish, flaxseeds, and walnuts), herbs (such as turmeric, ginger, and rosemary), and plenty of colorful fruits and vegetables.

Certain teas like dandelion root, green tea, ginger tea, and milk thistle can support liver function and enhance detoxification.

Warm lemon water in the morning can stimulate digestion and promote a gentle detox effect.

Superfoods like chlorella, spirulina, wheatgrass, and cilantro help bind heavy metals and other toxins in the body, supporting elimination through detox pathways.

Adding a green smoothie with some of these superfoods can enhance your body's natural cleansing processes.

Consistent physical activity not only helps promote sweat production but also enhances circulation, digestion, and oxygen flow, which support the body's detox systems.

Even light exercises like stretching, walking, or yoga can be beneficial for daily detoxification.

Breakfast Recipes

Coconut Chia Seed Pudding

Ingredients

- 3 tbsp chia seeds
- 1 cup coconut milk
- 1 tsp honey or maple syrup (optional)
- 1 tbsp shredded coconut

Other Info

Nutrition (per serving):

- Calories: 200
- Healthy Fats: 12g
- Fiber: 8g
- Protein: 5g
- Servings: 1
- Cooking Time: 5 minutes (plus refrigeration)

Directions

1. Mix chia seeds and coconut milk in a jar.
2. Add honey if using, and stir well.
3. Refrigerate overnight or for at least 2 hours until thickened.
4. Before serving, top with shredded coconut.
5. Stir and enjoy a creamy, nutritious breakfast.
6. Serve chilled.

Avocado and Tomato Breakfast Sandwich

Ingredients

- 1 slice whole-grain bread
- 1/2 avocado, mashed
- 1 small tomato, sliced
- A pinch of salt and pepper

Other Info

Nutrition (per serving):

- Calories: 180
- Healthy Fats: 10g
- Fiber: 6g
- Protein: 4g
- Servings: 1
- Cooking Time: 5 minutes

Directions

1. Toast the whole-grain bread until golden.
2. Spread mashed avocado on the toast.
3. Layer with tomato slices.
4. Sprinkle with salt and pepper.
5. Optionally, add fresh basil leaves for extra flavor.
6. Serve immediately as a refreshing breakfast sandwich.

Berry and Spinach Smoothie

Ingredients

- 1/2 cup mixed berries (frozen or fresh)
- A handful of fresh spinach
- 1/2 banana
- 1 cup almond milk

Other Info

Nutrition (per serving):

- Calories: 150
- Fiber: 5g
- Vitamin C: High
- Protein: 3g
- Servings: 1
- Cooking Time: 5 minutes

Directions

1. Add berries, spinach, banana, and almond milk to a blender.
2. Blend until smooth and creamy.
3. Pour into a glass.
4. Serve immediately for a nutrient-packed breakfast.
5. Optionally, add a few ice cubes for a chilled smoothie.
6. Sip slowly and enjoy.

Warm Apple Cinnamon Oatmeal

Ingredients

- 1/2 cup rolled oats
- 1 cup water or almond milk
- 1/2 apple, diced
- 1/2 tsp cinnamon

Other Info

Nutrition (per serving):

- Calories: 180
- Fiber: 6g
- Healthy Carbs: 32g
- Protein: 4g
- Servings: 1
- Cooking Time: 10 minutes

Directions

1. Bring water or almond milk to a boil in a pot.
2. Add oats and diced apple, cooking for 5 minutes until thickened.
3. Stir in cinnamon.
4. Serve warm, optionally topped with a sprinkle of nuts or seeds.
5. Sweeten with a drizzle of honey if desired.
6. Enjoy a comforting, balanced breakfast.

Scrambled Tofu Breakfast Bowl

Ingredients

- 1/2 cup firm tofu, crumbled
- 1/4 bell pepper, diced
- 1/4 onion, chopped
- 1 tsp olive oil
- A pinch of turmeric, salt, and pepper

Other Info

Nutrition (per serving):

- Calories: 160
- Protein: 9g
- Healthy Fats: 7g
- Fiber: 3g
- Servings: 1
- Cooking Time: 10 minutes

Directions

1. Heat olive oil in a pan over medium heat.
2. Add bell pepper and onion; sauté until softened.
3. Stir in crumbled tofu and season with turmeric, salt, and pepper.
4. Cook for 3-4 minutes until heated through.
5. Serve warm as a protein-rich breakfast bowl.
6. Optionally, top with fresh herbs.

Lunch Recipes

Lentil and Carrot Salad

Ingredients

- 1/2 cup cooked lentils
- 1 carrot, shredded
- 1 tbsp olive oil
- 1 tsp lemon juice
- A pinch of salt and pepper

Other Info

Nutrition (per serving):

- Calories: 180
- Protein: 8g
- Fiber: 8g
- Healthy Fats: 7g
- Servings: 1
- Cooking Time: 10 minutes

Directions

1. In a bowl, combine cooked lentils and shredded carrot.
2. Drizzle with olive oil and lemon juice.
3. Season with salt and pepper.
4. Mix well and let sit for 5 minutes to blend flavors.
5. Serve chilled or at room temperature.
6. Optionally, add parsley for extra flavor.

Quinoa and Cucumber Wrap

Ingredients

- 1 whole wheat tortilla
- 1/2 cup cooked quinoa
- 1/4 cucumber, sliced
- 1 tbsp hummus
- A pinch of salt and pepper

Other Info

Nutrition (per serving):

- Calories: 220
- Protein: 7g
- Fiber: 6g
- Healthy Fats: 5g
- Servings: 1
- Cooking Time: 5 minutes

Directions

1. Lay tortilla flat and spread hummus evenly over it.
2. Add cooked quinoa and sliced cucumber on top.
3. Season with salt and pepper.
4. Roll the tortilla tightly into a wrap.
5. Cut in half and serve immediately.
6. Enjoy with a side of fresh greens if desired.

Sautéed Broccoli and Chickpeas

Ingredients

- 1 cup broccoli florets
- 1/2 cup canned chickpeas (drained and rinsed)
- 1 tbsp olive oil
- A pinch of garlic powder, salt, and pepper

Other Info

Nutrition (per serving):

- Calories: 190
- Protein: 7g
- Fiber: 7g
- Healthy Fats: 8g
- Servings: 1
- Cooking Time: 10 minutes

Directions

1. Heat olive oil in a pan over medium heat.
2. Add broccoli and sauté for 3-4 minutes.
3. Stir in chickpeas and season with garlic powder, salt, and pepper.
4. Cook for another 3 minutes until broccoli is tender.
5. Serve warm as a protein-packed lunch.
6. Optionally, garnish with lemon zest.

Spinach and White Bean Salad

Ingredients

- 1 cup fresh spinach leaves
- 1/4 cup canned white beans (drained and rinsed)
- 1 tbsp olive oil
- A splash of apple cider vinegar
- Salt and pepper to taste

Other Info

Nutrition (per serving):

- Calories: 160
- Protein: 6g
- Fiber: 5g
- Healthy Fats: 9g
- Servings: 1
- Cooking Time: 5 minutes

Directions

1. Place spinach in a bowl and top with white beans.
2. Drizzle olive oil and apple cider vinegar over the salad.
3. Season with salt and pepper.
4. Toss gently to coat all ingredients.
5. Let sit for 2-3 minutes to blend flavors.
6. Serve as a light, refreshing lunch.

Sweet Potato and Red Bell Pepper Sauté

Ingredients

- 1/2 sweet potato, diced
- 1/2 red bell pepper, sliced
- 1 tsp coconut oil
- A pinch of cumin, salt, and pepper

Other Info

Nutrition (per serving):

- Calories: 170
- Fiber: 5g
- Healthy Fats: 4g
- Vitamin A: High
- Servings: 1
- Cooking Time: 15 minutes

Directions

1. Heat coconut oil in a pan over medium heat.
2. Add diced sweet potato and cook for 5-7 minutes until slightly tender.
3. Stir in red bell pepper and season with cumin, salt, and pepper.
4. Sauté for another 3-4 minutes until both vegetables are cooked.
5. Serve warm as a nutritious lunch option.
6. Pair with a side of mixed greens if desired.

Dinner

Recipes

Baked Lemon Dill Salmon

Ingredients

- 1 salmon fillet (about 4 oz)
- Juice of 1/2 lemon
- 1 tbsp olive oil
- Fresh dill, chopped
- Salt and pepper to taste

Other Info

Nutrition (per serving):

- Calories: 250
- Protein: 22g
- Healthy Fats: 14g
- Omega-3 Fatty Acids: High
- Servings: 1
- Cooking Time: 15 minutes

Directions

1. Preheat oven to 375°F (190°C).
2. Place salmon on a baking dish and drizzle with lemon juice and olive oil.
3. Season with salt, pepper, and dill.
4. Bake for 12-15 minutes until salmon is cooked through.
5. Serve warm with a side of steamed veggies.
6. Optionally, garnish with extra lemon slices.

Chickpea and Spinach Stir-Fry

Ingredients

- 1/2 cup canned chickpeas (drained and rinsed)
- 1 cup fresh spinach leaves
- 1 garlic clove, minced
- 1 tbsp olive oil
- A pinch of salt and pepper

Other Info

Nutrition (per serving):

- Calories: 180
- Protein: 7g
- Fiber: 6g
- Healthy Fats: 7g
- Servings: 1
- Cooking Time: 10 minutes

Directions

1. Heat olive oil in a pan over medium heat.
2. Add minced garlic and sauté until fragrant (about 1 minute).
3. Add chickpeas and cook for 3-4 minutes until slightly browned.
4. Stir in spinach and cook until wilted.
5. Season with salt and pepper.
6. Serve warm as a simple, nutrient-rich dinner.

Roasted Veggie Bowl

Ingredients

- 1/2 zucchini, sliced
- 1/2 bell pepper, diced
- 1/2 red onion, chopped
- 1 tbsp olive oil
- A pinch of salt, pepper, and thyme

Other Info

Nutrition (per serving):

- Calories: 150
- Fiber: 5g
- Healthy Fats: 8g
- Vitamin C: High
- Servings: 1
- Cooking Time: 25 minutes

Directions

1. Preheat oven to 400°F (200°C).
2. Toss all veggies with olive oil, salt, pepper, and thyme.
3. Spread evenly on a baking sheet.
4. Roast for 20-25 minutes until tender and slightly browned.
5. Serve as a warm dinner bowl.
6. Optionally, add a side of quinoa or brown rice.

Turkey and Sweet Potato Skillet

Ingredients

- 1/2 cup ground turkey
- 1 small sweet potato, diced
- 1/4 onion, chopped
- 1 tbsp olive oil
- A pinch of cumin, salt, and pepper

Other Info

Nutrition (per serving):

- Calories: 230
- Protein: 20g
- Healthy Fats: 8g
- Fiber: 4g
- Servings: 1
- Cooking Time: 15 minutes

Directions

1. Heat olive oil in a skillet over medium heat.
2. Add onion and sweet potato; cook for 5-7 minutes until slightly tender.
3. Stir in ground turkey and season with cumin, salt, and pepper.
4. Cook for 5-7 minutes until turkey is browned and cooked through.
5. Stir occasionally to prevent sticking.
6. Serve warm as a protein-rich, balanced dinner.

Garlic Shrimp with Asparagus

Ingredients

- 8-10 shrimp, peeled and deveined
- 1 cup asparagus spears, trimmed
- 1 garlic clove, minced
- 1 tbsp olive oil
- A pinch of salt and pepper

Other Info

Nutrition (per serving):

- Calories: 200
- Protein: 18g
- Healthy Fats: 9g
- Fiber: 3g
- Servings: 1
- Cooking Time: 10 minutes

Directions

1. Heat olive oil in a pan over medium heat.
2. Add minced garlic and sauté for 1 minute.
3. Add shrimp and asparagus to the pan.
4. Cook for 3-4 minutes until shrimp is pink and asparagus is tender.
5. Season with salt and pepper.
6. Serve immediately for a fresh, light dinner.

Snacks

Recipes

Apple Walnut Bites

Ingredients

- 1 apple, sliced
- 1 tbsp walnuts, chopped
- 1/2 tsp cinnamon
- A squeeze of lemon juice

Other Info

Nutrition (per serving):

- Calories: 120
- Fiber: 4g
- Healthy Fats: 7g
- Vitamin C: Moderate
- Servings: 1
- Cooking Time: 5 minutes

Directions

1. Slice apple and arrange on a plate.
2. Squeeze lemon juice over the slices to prevent browning.
3. Sprinkle chopped walnuts and cinnamon on top.
4. Let sit for a minute for flavors to blend.
5. Serve as a crunchy, sweet snack.
6. Enjoy immediately for the best texture.

Roasted Edamame

Ingredients

- 1/2 cup shelled edamame (fresh or frozen)
- 1 tsp olive oil
- A pinch of sea salt and pepper

Other Info

Nutrition (per serving):

- Calories: 100
- Protein: 8g
- Fiber: 4g
- Healthy Fats: 3g
- Servings: 1
- Cooking Time: 15 minutes

Directions

1. Preheat oven to 375°F (190°C).
2. Toss edamame with olive oil, salt, and pepper.
3. Spread evenly on a baking sheet.
4. Roast for 15 minutes until crispy, stirring halfway through.
5. Let cool slightly before serving.
6. Enjoy warm or at room temperature.

Banana Almond Butter Rounds

Ingredients

- 1 banana, sliced into rounds
- 1 tbsp almond butter
- A sprinkle of chia seeds (optional)

Other Info

Nutrition (per serving):

- Calories: 140
- Healthy Fats: 7g
- Fiber: 4g
- Potassium: High
- Servings: 1
- Cooking Time: 5 minutes

Directions

1. Arrange banana slices on a plate.
2. Spread a little almond butter on each slice.
3. Optionally, sprinkle with chia seeds for crunch.
4. Let sit for a minute to allow flavors to meld.
5. Enjoy as a quick, energy-boosting snack.
6. Best served immediately for freshness.

Carrot and Hummus Sticks

Ingredients

- 1 large carrot, cut into sticks
- 2 tbsp hummus
- A pinch of paprika (optional)

Other Info

Nutrition (per serving):

- Calories: 90
- Fiber: 4g
- Healthy Fats: 4g
- Vitamin A: High
- Servings: 1
- Cooking Time: 5 minutes

Directions

1. Cut carrot into sticks or thin strips.
2. Serve with a side of hummus for dipping.
3. Optionally, sprinkle hummus with paprika for added flavor.
4. Arrange carrot sticks neatly on a plate.
5. Enjoy as a refreshing and savory snack.
6. Perfect for a quick and healthy treat.

Mixed Berry Yogurt Bowl

Ingredients

- 1/2 cup plain Greek yogurt
- 1/4 cup mixed berries (blueberries, raspberries)
- 1 tsp flaxseeds
- A drizzle of honey (optional)

Other Info

Nutrition (per serving):

- Calories: 120
- Protein: 8g
- Fiber: 3g
- Healthy Fats: 3g
- Servings: 1
- Cooking Time: 5 minutes

Directions

1. Scoop yogurt into a small bowl.
2. Top with mixed berries and flaxseeds.
3. Drizzle with honey if you prefer a touch of sweetness.
4. Stir gently or leave layered for a pretty presentation.
5. Enjoy immediately as a protein-packed, refreshing snack.
6. Perfect for a morning or afternoon boost.

WEEK 4: HOW TO MAINTAIN BALANCE CORTISOL LEVELS

To maintain balanced cortisol levels, it's important to incorporate lifestyle habits that promote a healthy stress response, proper rest, and balanced nutrition. Here are some practical steps to help you achieve and sustain optimal cortisol balance:

1. Prioritize Quality Sleep

Establish a consistent sleep schedule: Go to bed and wake up at the same time each day to regulate your body's natural circadian rhythm, which plays a key role in cortisol production.

Create a calming bedtime routine: Avoid screens, caffeine, and heavy meals before bedtime; instead, engage in relaxing activities like reading, warm baths, or meditation.

Aim for 7-9 hours of sleep per night to prevent cortisol spikes caused by sleep deprivation.

2. Manage Stress Levels Effectively

Incorporate mindfulness practices: Techniques like meditation, deep breathing, progressive muscle relaxation, and yoga have been proven to help reduce stress and balance cortisol.

Daily relaxation breaks: Even taking a few minutes daily to focus on your breath, stretch, or relax can help control cortisol production.

Time in nature: Spending time outdoors, going for walks, and enjoying nature can naturally lower stress levels and improve your mood.

3. Eat a Balanced, Nutrient-Dense Diet

Consume whole foods: A diet rich in vegetables, fruits, whole grains, lean proteins, and healthy fats (like omega-3s) can help stabilize blood sugar levels and support balanced cortisol.

Eat regularly: Have balanced meals and snacks throughout the day to prevent blood sugar dips, which can trigger cortisol spikes. Don't skip meals, and ensure that you include complex carbohydrates, proteins, and healthy fats in every meal.

Limit stimulants: Reduce caffeine, processed foods, and refined sugars that can disrupt cortisol regulation and blood sugar balance.

4. Engage in Regular Physical Activity

Moderate-intensity exercise: Regular physical activity like walking, swimming, yoga, dancing, and strength training can help balance cortisol and reduce stress.

Avoid over-exercising: Excessive or intense workouts can lead to elevated cortisol levels, so focus on moderate exercise for at least 150 minutes per week. Listen to your body and take rest days when needed.

Mindful movement: Practices like tai chi and gentle yoga can help reduce cortisol and improve overall well-being without stressing the body.

5. Stay Hydrated

Proper hydration is essential for optimal cortisol regulation. Drinking 8-10 glasses of water daily can support kidney function and overall hormone balance.

Include hydrating foods in your diet, such as fruits, vegetables, and herbal teas, to support overall hydration.

6. Cultivate Healthy Relationships and Social Connections

Spend time with loved ones: Positive social interactions, laughter, and emotional support can improve mood and reduce stress, lowering cortisol levels.

Practice gratitude and positivity: Focusing on positive thoughts, writing gratitude lists, and engaging in uplifting conversations can help reduce stress and improve overall emotional well-being.

7. Establish Work-Life Balance

Set healthy boundaries: Balance work, personal time, and self-care to avoid burnout and chronic stress, which can elevate cortisol.

Manage your time effectively: Use organizational tools like planners, to-do lists, and calendars to manage daily tasks and avoid overwhelming stress.

Take regular breaks during work or stressful tasks to allow your mind to reset and lower cortisol levels.

8. Use Adaptogens and Herbal Support (If Needed)

Adaptogenic herbs like ashwagandha, rhodiola, holy basil, and ginseng can help support adrenal health and regulate cortisol levels.

Herbal teas like chamomile, lavender, and green tea can promote relaxation and balance cortisol. Consult with a healthcare provider before starting any herbal supplements.

9. Practice Self-Compassion and Mindfulness

Self-compassion: Accepting that you don't need to be perfect and allowing yourself to make mistakes can ease mental stress and prevent overproduction of cortisol.

Mindful activities: Engage in hobbies and activities that you enjoy, such as drawing, cooking, gardening, or playing a musical instrument, to keep stress levels low.

10. Limit Exposure to Blue Light in the Evening

Avoid screens before bed: Exposure to blue light from phones, computers, and TVs can interfere with melatonin production and disrupt cortisol balance.

Use blue light filters or glasses: If screen time is unavoidable, using filters or glasses that block blue light can help maintain healthy cortisol and melatonin levels for better sleep.

11. Keep Blood Sugar Balanced

Eat balanced meals with proteins, healthy fats, and complex carbohydrates to prevent blood sugar dips and spikes, which can trigger cortisol.

Avoid sugary snacks and refined carbohydrates that lead to blood sugar crashes and can disrupt cortisol production.

12. Take Breaks to Reset the Nervous System

Engage in activities like stretching, breathing exercises, listening to music, or taking short naps throughout the day to help your nervous system relax and support cortisol balance.
Mindful pauses, even for a few minutes, can make a big difference in how your body handles stress.

By making small, consistent lifestyle changes, you can effectively maintain balanced cortisol levels, supporting better health, emotional well-being, and a more resilient response to life's stressors.

Breakfast Recipes

Almond Coconut Oatmeal

Ingredients

- 1/2 cup rolled oats
- 1 cup almond milk
- 1 tbsp shredded coconut
- 1 tbsp almond slivers
- A pinch of cinnamon

Other Info

Nutrition (per serving):

- Calories: 200
- Healthy Fats: 8g
- Fiber: 5g
- Protein: 6g
- Servings: 1
- Cooking Time: 10 minutes

Directions

1. In a pot, bring almond milk to a boil.
2. Stir in oats and reduce heat; cook for 5 minutes until thickened.
3. Stir in shredded coconut and cinnamon.
4. Serve warm, topped with almond slivers.
5. Optionally, sweeten with a touch of honey.
6. Enjoy as a comforting, nutrient-rich breakfast.

Strawberry Banana Smoothie Bowl

Ingredients

- 1/2 banana
- 1/2 cup strawberries (fresh or frozen)
- 1/2 cup Greek yogurt
- 1 tbsp chia seeds

Other Info

Nutrition (per serving):

- Calories: 180
- Protein: 8g
- Fiber: 5g
- Vitamin C: High
- Servings: 1
- Cooking Time: 5 minutes

Directions

1. Blend banana, strawberries, and yogurt until smooth.
2. Pour mixture into a bowl.
3. Top with chia seeds for crunch.
4. Optionally, add extra sliced strawberries or banana on top.
5. Serve immediately for a cool and refreshing breakfast.
6. Enjoy with a spoon!

Savory Avocado and Egg Toast

Ingredients

- 1 slice whole grain bread
- 1/2 ripe avocado, mashed
- 1 egg (boiled or poached)
- A pinch of salt, pepper, and paprika

Other Info

Nutrition (per serving):

- Calories: 220
- Protein: 9g
- Healthy Fats: 14g
- Fiber: 5g
- Servings: 1
- Cooking Time: 8 minutes

Directions

1. Toast the bread until crisp.
2. Spread mashed avocado on the toast.
3. Top with the egg, sliced or halved.
4. Season with salt, pepper, and paprika.
5. Serve immediately for a protein-rich start to your day.
6. Enjoy with a side of fresh greens if desired.

Pear and Cinnamon Yogurt Parfait

Ingredients

- 1/2 cup plain Greek yogurt
- 1 small pear, diced
- 1 tsp ground cinnamon
- 1 tbsp walnuts, chopped

Other Info

Nutrition (per serving):

- Calories: 180
- Protein: 10g
- Fiber: 4g
- Healthy Fats: 7g
- Servings: 1
- Cooking Time: 5 minutes

Directions

1. Scoop Greek yogurt into a bowl or glass.
2. Layer with diced pear on top.
3. Sprinkle with cinnamon.
4. Top with chopped walnuts for crunch.
5. Serve immediately for a sweet and satisfying breakfast.
6. Stir lightly if preferred.

Tomato Basil Breakfast Scramble

Ingredients

- 2 eggs, whisked
- 1/4 cup cherry tomatoes, halved
- Fresh basil leaves, chopped
- 1 tsp olive oil
- Salt and pepper to taste

Other Info

Nutrition (per serving):

- Calories: 150
- Protein: 12g
- Healthy Fats: 9g
- Vitamin A: High
- Servings: 1
- Cooking Time: 8 minutes

Directions

1. Heat olive oil in a pan over medium heat.
2. Add cherry tomatoes and sauté until slightly soft.
3. Pour in whisked eggs and scramble until cooked through.
4. Stir in fresh basil just before removing from heat.
5. Season with salt and pepper.
6. Serve warm as a flavorful and simple breakfast.

Lunch

Recipes

Grilled Veggie and Hummus Wrap

Ingredients

- 1 whole wheat tortilla
- 1/4 zucchini, sliced
- 1/4 red bell pepper, sliced
- 2 tbsp hummus
- 1 tsp olive oil

Other Info

Nutrition (per serving):

- Calories: 220
- Protein: 7g
- Fiber: 6g
- Healthy Fats: 8g
- Servings: 1
- Cooking Time: 10 minutes

Directions

1. Heat olive oil in a pan and grill zucchini and red bell pepper until slightly charred.
2. Spread hummus over the tortilla.
3. Place grilled veggies on top and roll up tightly.
4. Cut in half and serve warm or at room temperature.
5. Enjoy as a quick, filling lunch.
6. Optional: add greens for extra crunch.

Quinoa and Bean Salad

Ingredients

- 1/2 cup cooked quinoa
- 1/4 cup black beans (drained and rinsed)
- 1/4 cup cherry tomatoes, halved
- 1 tbsp olive oil
- A splash of lime juice

Other Info

Nutrition (per serving):

- Calories: 230
- Protein: 8g
- Fiber: 7g
- Healthy Fats: 8g
- Servings: 1
- Cooking Time: 10 minutes

Directions

1. Mix cooked quinoa, black beans, and cherry tomatoes in a bowl.
2. Drizzle with olive oil and lime juice.
3. Stir to combine all ingredients well.
4. Let sit for 5 minutes for flavors to meld.
5. Serve chilled or at room temperature.
6. Optional: garnish with cilantro.

Spinach and Avocado Salad

Ingredients

- 1 cup fresh spinach leaves
- 1/2 avocado, diced
- 1 tbsp sunflower seeds
- 1 tbsp olive oil
- A squeeze of lemon juice

Other Info

Nutrition (per serving):

- Calories: 180
- Fiber: 6g
- Healthy Fats: 14g
- Protein: 4g
- Servings: 1
- Cooking Time: 5 minutes

Directions

1. Place spinach leaves in a bowl.
2. Top with diced avocado and sunflower seeds.
3. Drizzle with olive oil and lemon juice.
4. Toss gently to coat the salad evenly.
5. Serve fresh and enjoy.
6. Optionally, add a pinch of salt and pepper.

Tomato and Basil Lentil Soup

Ingredients

- 1/2 cup cooked lentils
- 1 cup vegetable broth
- 1/4 cup diced tomatoes
- Fresh basil, chopped
- A pinch of salt and pepper

Other Info

Nutrition (per serving):

- Calories: 150
- Protein: 8g
- Fiber: 6g
- Vitamin A: High
- Servings: 1
- Cooking Time: 10 minutes

Directions

1. In a pot, bring vegetable broth and diced tomatoes to a boil.
2. Add cooked lentils and reduce heat to simmer for 5 minutes.
3. Stir in chopped basil and season with salt and pepper.
4. Simmer for another 2 minutes.
5. Serve warm as a comforting lunch.
6. Optionally, add a drizzle of olive oil on top.

Baked Sweet Potato with Tzatziki

Ingredients

- 1 small sweet potato
- 2 tbsp tzatziki sauce (store-bought or homemade)
- A pinch of salt
- A sprinkle of parsley (optional)

Other Info

Nutrition (per serving):

- Calories: 180
- Fiber: 4g
- Healthy Carbs: Moderate
- Protein: 3g
- Servings: 1
- Cooking Time: 35 minutes

Directions

1. Preheat oven to 400°F (200°C).
2. Pierce sweet potato with a fork and bake for 30-35 minutes until tender.
3. Slice open and sprinkle with salt.
4. Top with tzatziki sauce and parsley if using.
5. Serve warm as a savory, flavorful lunch.
6. Enjoy with a side of mixed greens if desired.

Dinner

Recipes

Lemon Herb Baked Chicken

Ingredients

- 1 chicken breast (4 oz)
- Juice of 1/2 lemon
- 1 tbsp olive oil
- Dried oregano, salt, and pepper to taste

Other Info

Nutrition (per serving):

- Calories: 220
- Protein: 26g
- Healthy Fats: 11g
- Vitamin C: Moderate
- Servings: 1
- Cooking Time: 25 minutes

Directions

1. Preheat oven to 375°F (190°C).
2. Marinate chicken with lemon juice, olive oil, oregano, salt, and pepper.
3. Place chicken on a baking dish and bake for 20-25 minutes until cooked through.
4. Let rest for a minute before slicing.
5. Serve warm with a side of steamed vegetables.
6. Optionally garnish with fresh herbs.

Veggie Stuffed Bell Peppers

Ingredients

- 1 bell pepper (any color)
- 1/2 cup cooked quinoa
- 1/4 cup black beans (drained and rinsed)
- 1 tbsp olive oil
- Salt and pepper to taste

Other Info

Nutrition (per serving):

- Calories: 200
- Protein: 7g
- Fiber: 6g
- Healthy Fats: 7g
- Servings: 1
- Cooking Time: 25 minutes

Directions

1. Preheat oven to 375°F (190°C).
2. Cut the top off the bell pepper, remove seeds, and set aside.
3. Mix quinoa, black beans, olive oil, salt, and pepper.
4. Stuff the bell pepper with the quinoa mixture.
5. Bake for 20-25 minutes until the pepper is tender.
6. Serve warm as a balanced, nutritious dinner.

Sautéed Shrimp with Garlic and Spinach

Ingredients

- 8 shrimp (peeled and deveined)
- 1 cup fresh spinach
- 1 garlic clove, minced
- 1 tbsp olive oil
- A pinch of salt and pepper

Other Info

Nutrition (per serving):

- Calories: 180
- Protein: 18g
- Healthy Fats: 9g
- Vitamin A: High
- Servings: 1
- Cooking Time: 10 minutes

Directions

1. Heat olive oil in a pan over medium heat.
2. Add garlic and sauté until fragrant.
3. Add shrimp and cook until pink (about 3-4 minutes).
4. Stir in spinach and sauté until wilted.
5. Season with salt and pepper before serving.
6. Enjoy with a side of brown rice or quinoa if desired.

Roasted Sweet Potato and Broccoli Plate

Ingredients

- 1 small sweet potato, diced
- 1 cup broccoli florets
- 1 tbsp olive oil
- A pinch of paprika, salt, and pepper

Other Info

Nutrition (per serving):

- Calories: 190
- Fiber: 7g
- Healthy Fats: 8g
- Vitamin A: High
- Servings: 1
- Cooking Time: 30 minutes

Directions

1. Preheat oven to 400°F (200°C).
2. Toss sweet potato and broccoli with olive oil, paprika, salt, and pepper.
3. Spread on a baking sheet in a single layer.
4. Roast for 25-30 minutes until tender and slightly crispy.
5. Stir halfway through for even cooking.
6. Serve warm as a hearty veggie dinner.

Tofu and Vegetable Stir-Fry

Ingredients

- 1/2 cup firm tofu, cubed
- 1/4 cup sliced carrots
- 1/4 cup sliced bell peppers
- 1 tbsp soy sauce or tamari
- 1 tsp sesame oil

Other Info

Nutrition (per serving):

- Calories: 160
- Protein: 10g
- Healthy Fats: 7g
- Fiber: 4g
- Servings: 1
- Cooking Time: 10 minutes

Directions

1. Heat sesame oil in a pan over medium heat.
2. Add tofu and sauté until golden brown (about 4 minutes).
3. Add carrots and bell peppers; stir-fry until slightly tender.
4. Drizzle soy sauce over the stir-fry.
5. Cook for another 2 minutes until vegetables are crisp-tender.
6. Serve immediately as a flavorful, plant-based dinner.

Snacks

Recipes

Cucumber and Dill Yogurt Dip

Ingredients

- 1/2 cucumber, sliced
- 1/4 cup plain Greek yogurt
- A pinch of dried dill
- A squeeze of lemon juice

Other Info

Nutrition (per serving):

- Calories: 70
- Protein: 5g
- Fiber: 1g
- Healthy Fats: 2g
- Servings: 1
- Cooking Time: 5 minutes

Directions

1. In a bowl, mix Greek yogurt, dill, and lemon juice.
2. Slice cucumber into thin rounds.
3. Serve cucumber slices with the yogurt dip on the side.
4. Enjoy as a light, refreshing snack.
5. Optionally, sprinkle yogurt with salt and pepper.
6. Perfect for a quick and cooling treat.

Almond and Blueberry Snack Mix

Ingredients

- 10 almonds
- 1/4 cup fresh blueberries
- A pinch of cinnamon

Other Info

Nutrition (per serving):

- Calories: 90
- Healthy Fats: 6g
- Fiber: 3g
- Vitamin C: Moderate
- Servings: 1
- Cooking Time: 2 minutes

Directions

1. Place almonds and blueberries in a small bowl.
2. Sprinkle with a pinch of cinnamon.
3. Mix gently to coat the almonds and berries.
4. Serve as a quick, antioxidant-rich snack.
5. Perfect for an on-the-go treat.
6. Optionally, pair with green tea.

Apple and Sunflower Seed Butter Slices

Ingredients

- 1 apple, sliced
- 1 tbsp sunflower seed butter

Other Info

Nutrition (per serving):

- Calories: 120
- Healthy Fats: 6g
- Fiber: 4g
- Protein: 2g
- Servings: 1
- Cooking Time: 3 minutes

Directions

1. Core and slice the apple into wedges.
2. Spread a thin layer of sunflower seed butter on each apple slice.
3. Arrange on a plate for easy snacking.
4. Enjoy as a sweet and savory combo.
5. Serve immediately to prevent apple browning.
6. Optionally, sprinkle with a pinch of cinnamon for extra flavor.

Carrot Sticks with Spicy Hummus

Ingredients

- 1 large carrot, cut into sticks
- 2 tbsp hummus
- A pinch of paprika or cayenne pepper

Other Info

Nutrition (per serving):

- Calories: 80
- Fiber: 3g
- Healthy Fats: 4g
- Protein: 2g
- Servings: 1
- Cooking Time: 5 minutes

Directions

1. Cut carrot into sticks for easy dipping.
2. Place hummus in a small bowl.
3. Sprinkle hummus with paprika or cayenne pepper for a spicy kick.
4. Serve carrot sticks with the hummus on the side.
5. Enjoy as a crunchy, flavorful snack.
6. Great for a quick, nutrient-rich pick-me-up.

Pear and Pumpkin Seed Bites

Ingredients

- 1 small pear, sliced
- 1 tbsp pumpkin seeds
- A drizzle of honey (optional)

Other Info

Nutrition (per serving):

- Calories: 100
- Fiber: 4g
- Healthy Fats: 4g
- Protein: 2g
- Servings: 1
- Cooking Time: 5 minutes

Directions

1. Slice pear into thin wedges.
2. Sprinkle pumpkin seeds over the pear slices.
3. Drizzle with a little honey if desired.
4. Arrange on a plate for a quick snack.
5. Serve immediately for the best freshness.
6. Optionally, add a sprinkle of cinnamon for extra flavor.

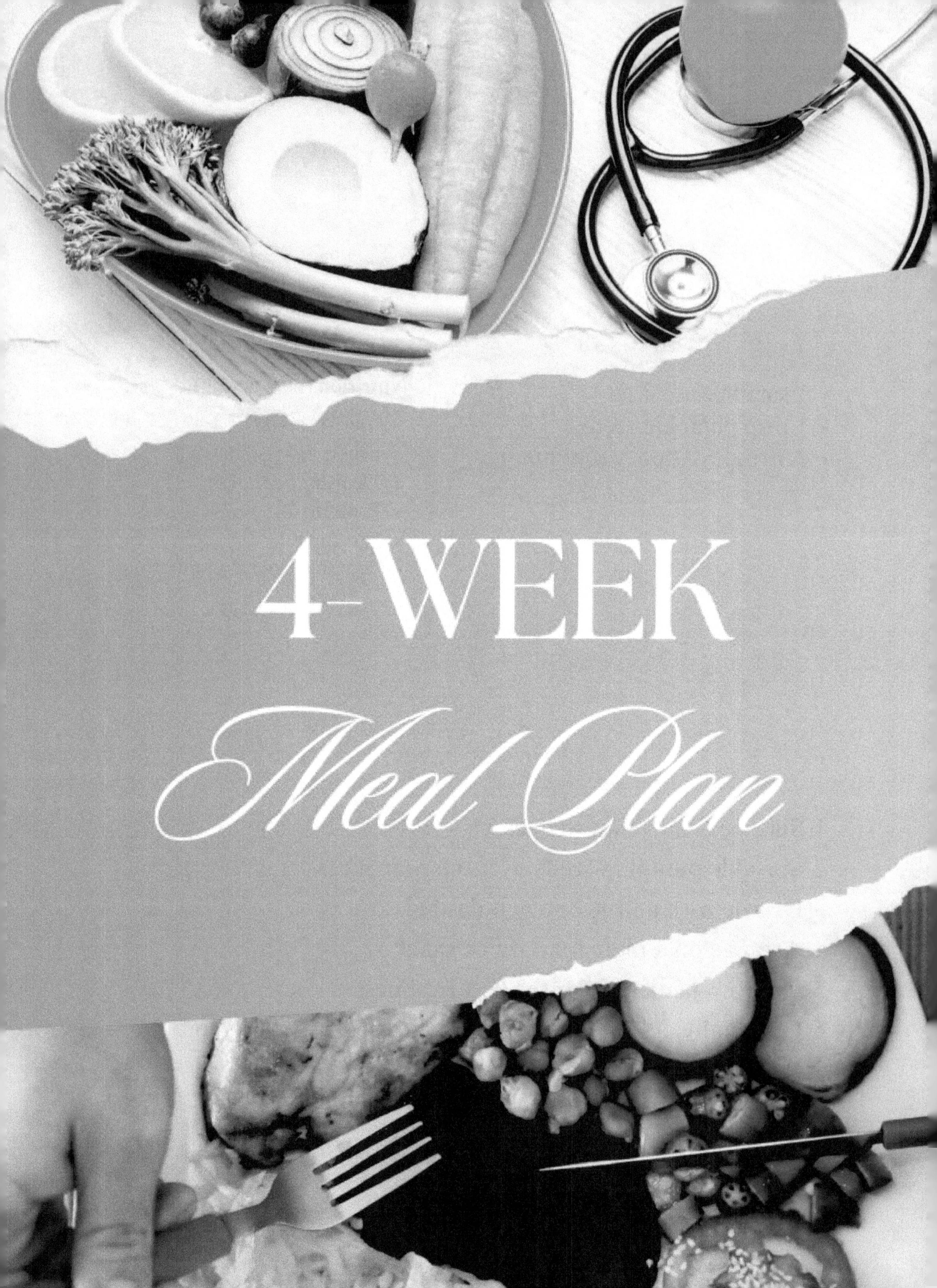

4-WEEK
Meal Plan

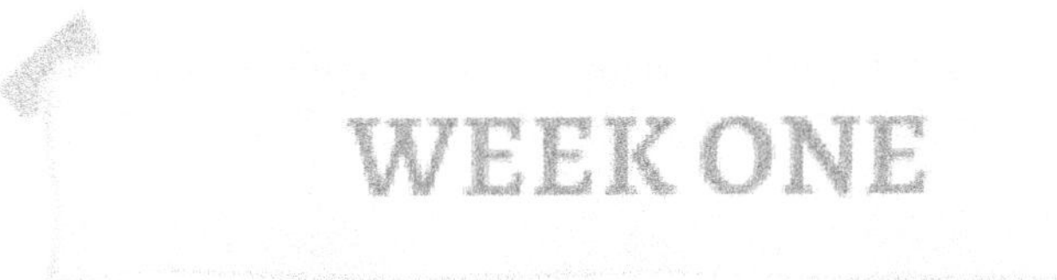

MONDAY

Breakfast: Avocado and Spinach Toast
Lunch: Quinoa and Chickpea Salad
Dinner: Baked Salmon with Asparagus

TUESDAY

Breakfast: Blueberry Almond Overnight Oats
Lunch: Turkey and Spinach Wrap
Dinner: Quinoa and Veggie Stuffed Peppers

WEDNESDAY

Breakfast: Greek Yogurt Parfait
Lunch: Lentil and Veggie Soup
Dinner: Lemon-Garlic Shrimp and Broccoli

THURSDAY

Breakfast: Banana and Chia Seed Smoothie
Lunch: Grilled Chicken and Avocado Salad
Dinner: Sweet Potato and Lentil Curry

FRIDAY

Breakfast: Scrambled Eggs with Tomato and Basil
Lunch: Veggie and Brown Rice Stir-Fry
Dinner: Zucchini Noodles with Pesto and Cherry Tomatoes

SATURDAY

Breakfast: Avocado and Spinach Toast
Lunch: Quinoa and Chickpea Salad
Dinner: Baked Salmon with Asparagus

SUNDAY

Breakfast: Blueberry Almond Overnight Oats
Lunch: Turkey and Spinach Wrap
Dinner: Quinoa and Veggie Stuffed Peppers

WEEK TWO

MONDAY

Breakfast: Berry and Nut Chia Pudding

Lunch: Mediterranean Chickpea Bowl

Dinner: Grilled Lemon Herb Chicken with Zucchini

TUESDAY

Breakfast: Banana Oat Pancakes

Lunch: Lentil and Avocado Lettuce Wraps

Dinner: Shrimp and Cauliflower Rice Stir-Fry

WEDNESDAY

Breakfast: Sweet Potato Breakfast Hash

Lunch: Brown Rice and Black Bean Bowl

Dinner: Baked Cod with Cherry Tomatoes and Basil

THURSDAY

Breakfast: Pear and Walnut Parfait

Lunch: Tuna and Spinach Salad

Dinner: Turkey and Veggie Skewers

FRIDAY

Breakfast: Berry and Nut Chia Pudding

Lunch: Mediterranean Chickpea Bowl

Dinner: Veggie and Tofu Stir-Fry

SATURDAY

Breakfast: Banana Oat Pancakes

Lunch: Lentil and Avocado Lettuce Wraps

Dinner: Grilled Lemon Herb Chicken with Zucchini

SUNDAY

Breakfast: Sweet Potato Breakfast Hash

Lunch: Brown Rice and Black Bean Bowl

Dinner: Shrimp and Cauliflower Rice Stir-Fry

WEEK THREE

MONDAY
Breakfast: Coconut Chia Seed Pudding
Lunch: Lentil and Carrot Salad
Dinner: Baked Lemon Dill Salmon

TUESDAY
Breakfast: Avocado and Tomato Breakfast Sandwich
Lunch: Quinoa and Cucumber Wrap
Dinner: Chickpea and Spinach Stir-Fry

WEDNESDAY
Breakfast: Berry and Spinach Smoothie
Lunch: Sautéed Broccoli and Chickpeas
Dinner: Roasted Veggie Bowl

THURSDAY
Breakfast: Warm Apple Cinnamon Oatmeal
Lunch: Spinach and White Bean Salad
Dinner: Turkey and Sweet Potato Skillet

FRIDAY
Breakfast: Scrambled Tofu Breakfast Bowl
Lunch: Sweet Potato and Red Bell Pepper Sauté
Dinner: Garlic Shrimp with Asparagus

SATURDAY
Breakfast: Coconut Chia Seed Pudding
Lunch: Lentil and Carrot Salad
Dinner: Baked Lemon Dill Salmon

SUNDAY
Breakfast: Avocado and Tomato Breakfast Sandwich
Lunch: Quinoa and Cucumber Wrap
Dinner: Chickpea and Spinach Stir-Fry

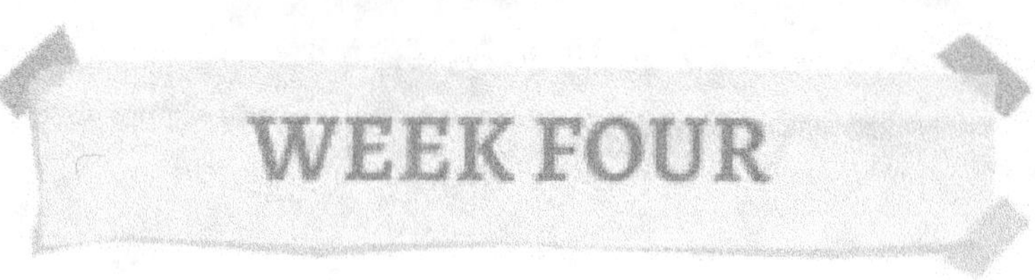

WEEK FOUR

MONDAY

Breakfast: Almond Coconut Oatmeal
Lunch: Grilled Veggie and Hummus Wrap
Dinner: Lemon Herb Baked Chicken

TUESDAY

Breakfast: Savory Avocado and Egg Toast
Lunch: Quinoa and Bean Salad
Dinner: Veggie Stuffed Bell Peppers

WEDNESDAY

Breakfast: Pear and Cinnamon Yogurt Parfait
Lunch: Spinach and Avocado Salad
Dinner: Sautéed Shrimp with Garlic and Spinach

THURSDAY

Breakfast: Tomato Basil Breakfast Scramble
Lunch: Tomato and Basil Lentil Soup
Dinner: Roasted Sweet Potato and Broccoli Plate

FRIDAY

Breakfast: Almond Coconut Oatmeal
Lunch: Baked Sweet Potato with Tzatziki
Dinner: Tofu and Vegetable Stir-Fry

SATURDAY

Breakfast: Savory Avocado and Egg Toast
Lunch: Grilled Veggie and Hummus Wrap
Dinner: Lemon Herb Baked Chicken

SUNDAY

Breakfast: Pear and Cinnamon Yogurt Parfait
Lunch: Quinoa and Bean Salad
Dinner: Veggie Stuffed Bell Peppers

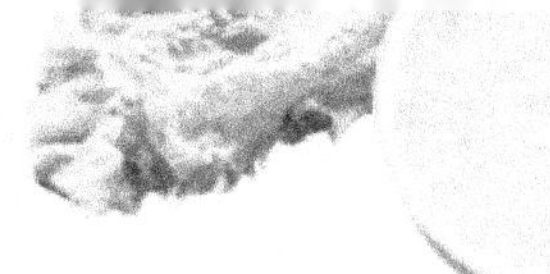

LIST OF INGREDIENTS

VEGETABLES

- Avocados
- Spinach
- Tomatoes
- Basil
- Asparagus
- Zucchini
- Sweet Potatoes
- Broccoli
- Cherry Tomatoes
- Bell Peppers (Red, Green, or Yellow)
- Cauliflower
- Carrots
- Cucumber
- Lettuce (for wraps)
- Kale
- Red Bell Pepper
- Garlic
- Onion
- White Beans
- Chickpeas
- Lentils
- Quinoa
- Tofu

FRUITS

- Blueberries
- Bananas
- Pears
- Apples
- Almonds
- Walnuts
- Berries (Mixed, Strawberries, Raspberries, etc.)
- Lemons
- Dates
- Coconut (shredded or flakes)
- Pumpkin Seeds

GRAINS & BREAD

- Whole Grain Bread (for toast and sandwiches)
- Brown Rice
- Oats (rolled or steel-cut)
- Quinoa
- Chia Seeds

LIST OF INGREDIENTS

PROTEIN

- Eggs
- Greek Yogurt
- Chicken Breasts (boneless, skinless)
- Turkey (ground or breast)
- Salmon (fillets)
- Cod (fillets)
- Shrimp
- Tofu
- Black Beans
- Tuna (canned in water or fresh)
- Edamame
- Almond Butter
- Sunflower Seed Butter

DAIRY

- Greek Yogurt (plain, unsweetened)
- Tzatziki Sauce
- Almond Milk or Coconut Milk (for chia pudding, smoothies, and oatmeal)

NUTS & SEEDS

- Almonds
- Pumpkin Seeds
- Sunflower Seeds
- Walnuts
- Chia Seeds
- Flaxseeds (optional for smoothies)

HERBS & SPICES

- Basil (fresh or dried)
- Cinnamon
- Dill
- Mint
- Lemon Zest
- Garlic Powder
- Cumin
- Salt (sea salt or kosher salt)
- Black Pepper
- Paprika (optional)
- Red Pepper Flakes (optional)

LIST OF INGREDIENTS

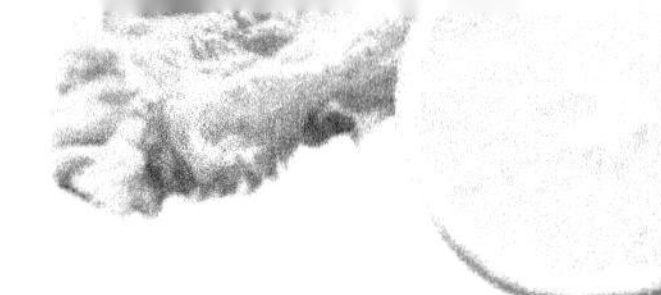

OILS & CONDIMENTS

- **Olive Oil (extra virgin for cooking and dressing)**
- **Pesto Sauce (for zucchini noodles)**
- **Hummus (for dips and wraps)**
- **Guacamole (for snacks or spreads)**
- **Dark Chocolate (optional for almond and chocolate mix)**

MISCELLANEOUS

- **Almond Butter (for snacks or toast)**
- **Almond Flour (optional for some recipes like pancakes)**
- **Energy Bites (almond date, nut-based)**
- **Nut Butter (almond or peanut, for snacks)**

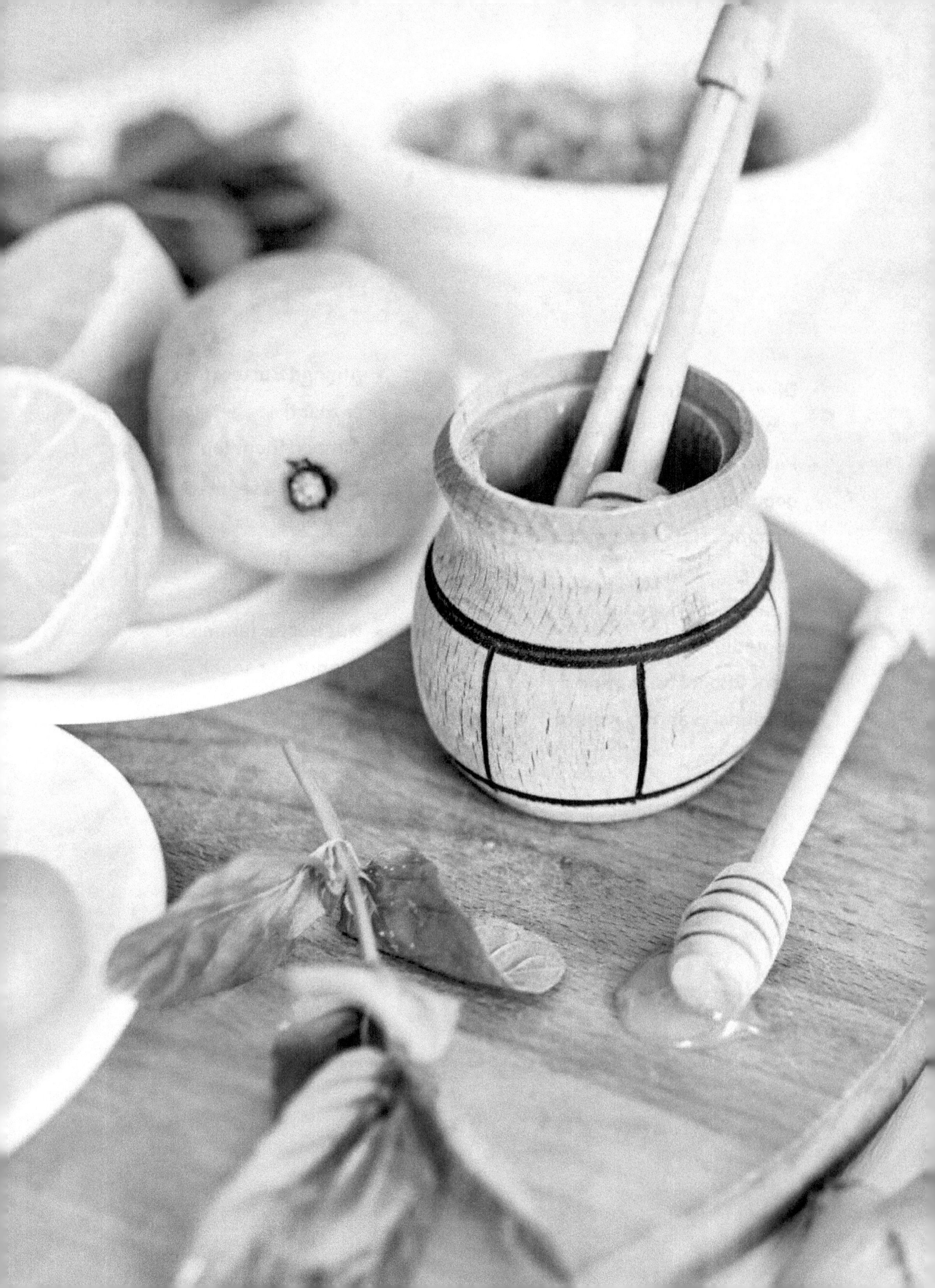

Conclusion

The Complete Cortisol Detox Diet Plan offers a powerful, holistic approach to reducing stress, balancing hormones, and enhancing overall well-being. By focusing on nutrient-dense meals, regular exercise, hydration, and self-care, this plan helps to naturally regulate cortisol levels, leading to improved mood, better sleep, and reduced anxiety.

The diet emphasizes whole foods like lean proteins, healthy fats, complex carbs, and fiber-rich vegetables, alongside mindful lifestyle practices that encourage relaxation, sleep quality, and emotional balance. By supporting the body's natural detoxification processes and reducing inflammation, this approach helps break the cycle of stress and restore the body's ability to cope effectively with daily pressures.

It's more than just a diet; it's a lifestyle shift towards sustained wellness. Adopting this plan can empower you to regain control of your health and find peace in your mind and body. Remember, every step you take towards better habits is a step towards a more balanced life. Start small—whether it's trying a new breakfast recipe, committing to a daily walk, or taking a few moments to breathe deeply.

Embrace the journey, stay consistent, and soon you'll experience the transformative power of a life lived in balance and harmony. Your best self is just one change away.

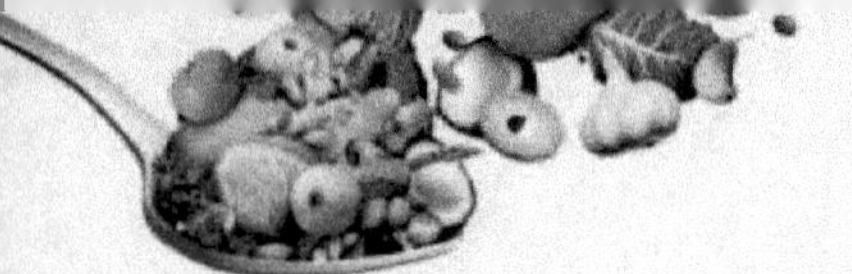

MEAL PLANNER

| WEEK OF: | MONTH: | YEAR: |

	BREAKFAST	LUNCH	DINNER	SNACK & FRUITS
MON				
TUE				
WED				
THU				
FRI				
SAT				
SUN				

NOTES

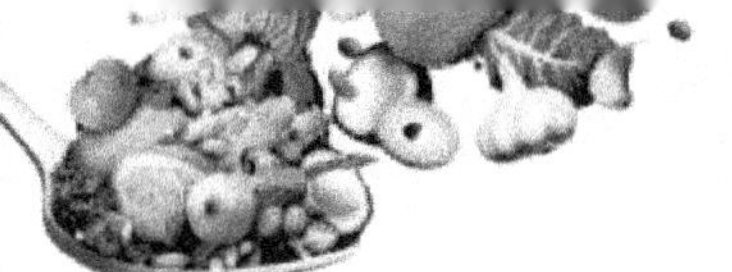

MEAL PLANNER

WEEK OF:	MONTH:	YEAR:

	BREAKFAST	LUNCH	DINNER	SNACK & FRUITS
MON				
TUE				
WED				
THU				
FRI				
SAT				
SUN				

NOTES

MEAL PLANNER

WEEK OF: MONTH: YEAR:

	BREAKFAST	LUNCH	DINNER	SNACK & FRUITS
MON				
TUE				
WED				
THU				
FRI				
SAT				
SUN				

NOTES

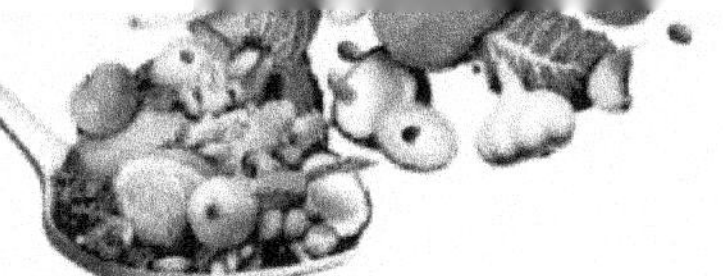

MEAL PLANNER

WEEK OF: MONTH: YEAR:

	BREAKFAST	LUNCH	DINNER	SNACK & FRUITS
MON				
TUE				
WED				
THU				
FRI				
SAT				
SUN				

NOTES

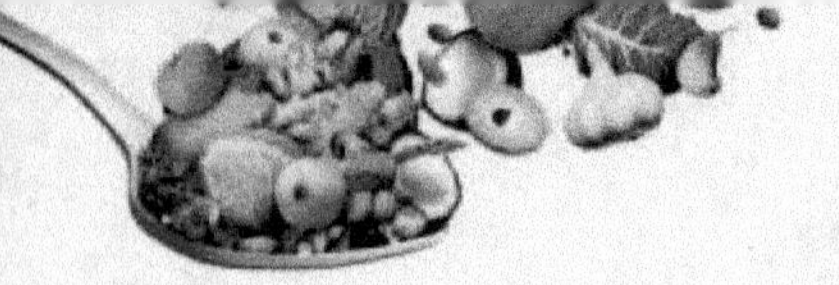

MEAL PLANNER

WEEK OF: MONTH: YEAR:

	BREAKFAST	LUNCH	DINNER	SNACK & FRUITS
MON				
TUE				
WED				
THU				
FRI				
SAT				
SUN				

NOTES

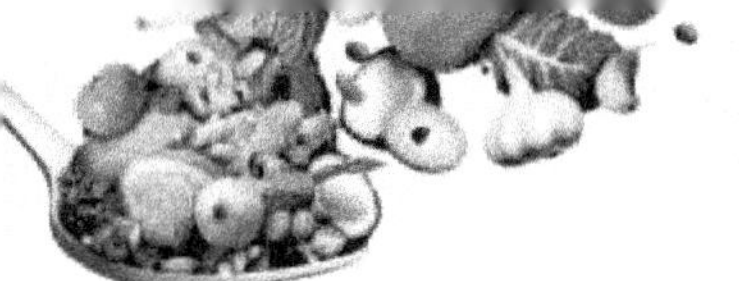

MEAL PLANNER

WEEK OF:	MONTH:	YEAR:

	BREAKFAST	LUNCH	DINNER	SNACK & FRUITS
MON				
TUE				
WED				
THU				
FRI				
SAT				
SUN				

NOTES

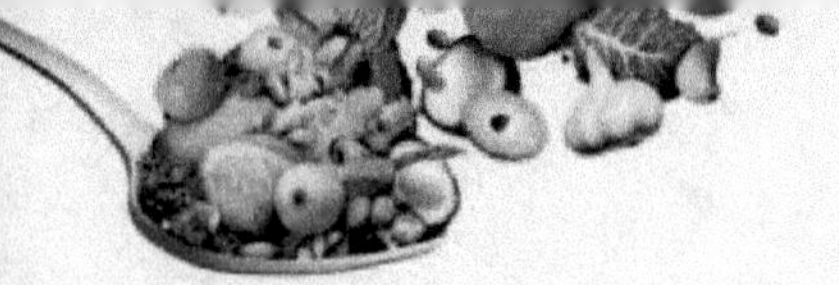

MEAL PLANNER

WEEK OF: MONTH: YEAR:

	BREAKFAST	LUNCH	DINNER	SNACK & FRUITS
MON				
TUE				
WED				
THU				
FRI				
SAT				
SUN				

NOTES

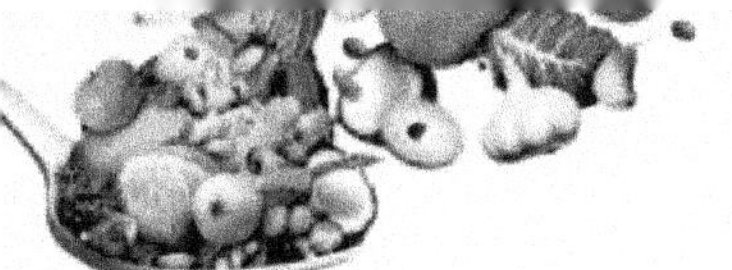

MEAL PLANNER

WEEK OF: MONTH: YEAR:

	BREAKFAST	LUNCH	DINNER	SNACK & FRUITS
MON				
TUE				
WED				
THU				
FRI				
SAT				
SUN				

NOTES

MEAL PLANNER

WEEK OF: MONTH: YEAR:

	BREAKFAST	LUNCH	DINNER	SNACK & FRUITS
MON				
TUE				
WED				
THU				
FRI				
SAT				
SUN				

NOTES

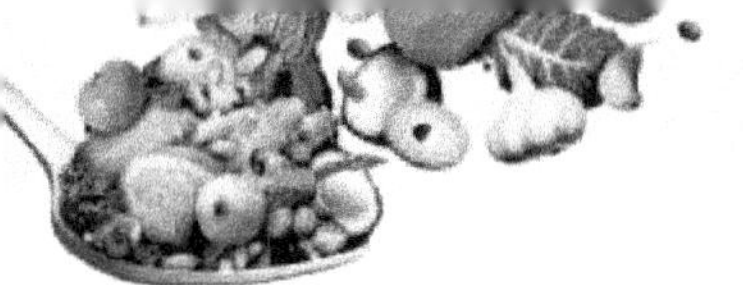

MEAL PLANNER

| WEEK OF: | | MONTH: | | YEAR: |

	BREAKFAST	LUNCH	DINNER	SNACK & FRUITS
MON				
TUE				
WED				
THU				
FRI				
SAT				
SUN				

NOTES

THANK YOU
FOR READING!

THANK YOU FOR PURCHASING THE COMPLETE CORTISOL DETOX DIET PLAN

I HOPE YOU FIND THE RECIPES BOTH ENJOYABLE AND HELPFUL ON YOUR CULINARY JOURNEY. YOUR FEEDBACK MEANS A LOT TO ME—PLEASE CONSIDER LEAVING AN HONEST REVIEW TO HELP OTHERS DISCOVER THE BOOK.

HAPPY COOKING

AMADA L. HEATH

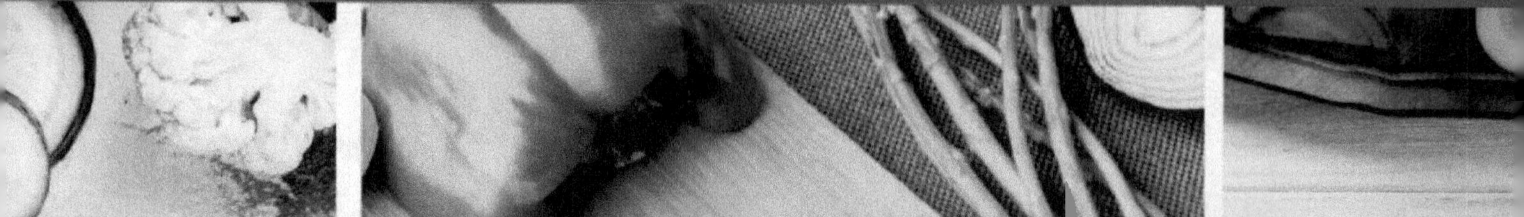

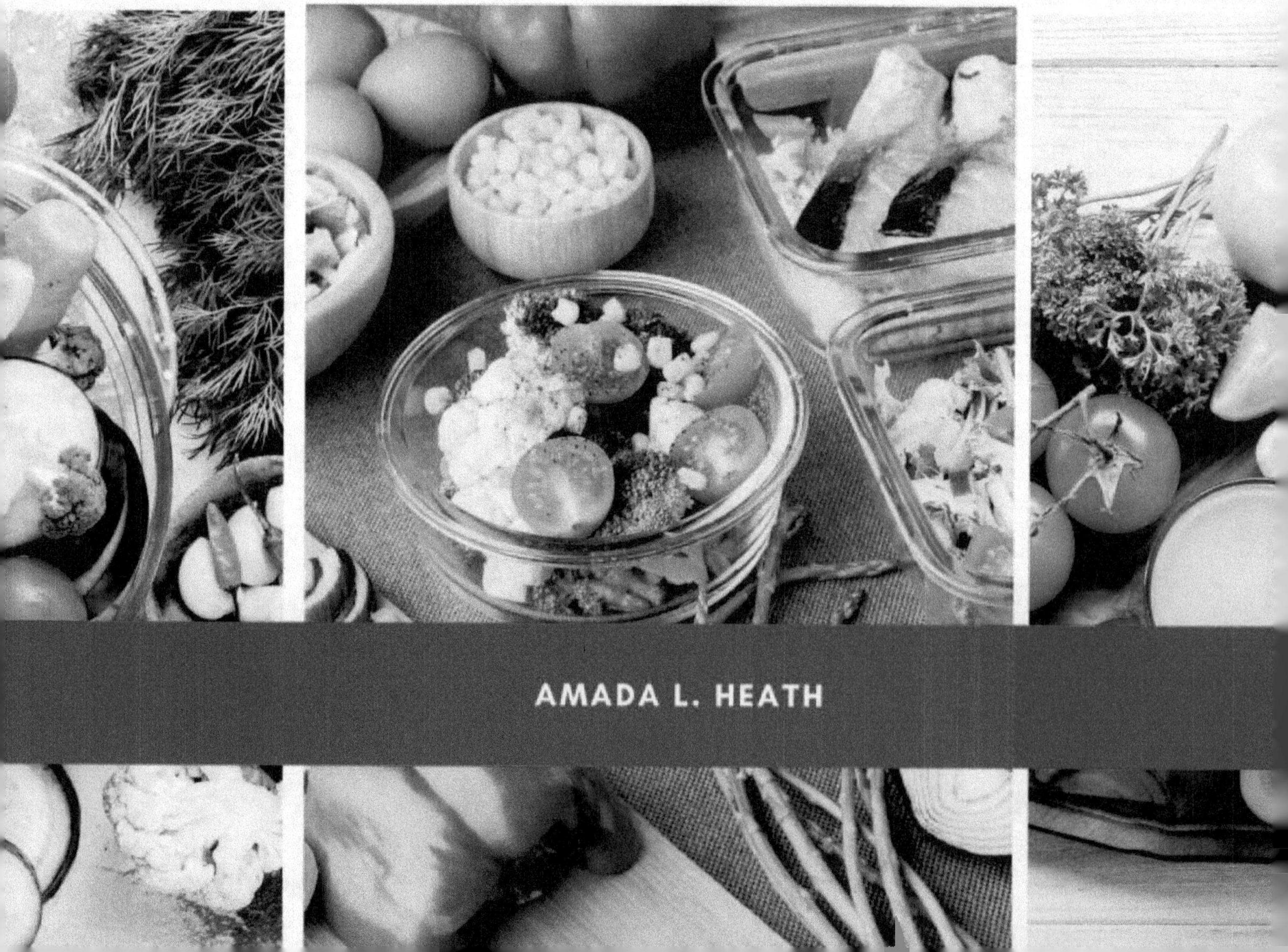